Praise for
The Heart of We

"*The Heart of Wellness* is a perfect blend ⟨ ▨ latest medical science. Dr. Chinnaiyan ha⟩ ▨ ▨ much needed template for the true application of Vedic sciences in integrative medicine. Kudos!"—Suhas Kshirsagar, BAMS (Bachelor of Ayurvedic Medicine and Surgery), MD, author of *Change Your Schedule Change Your Life* (Harper Collins, 2018)

"What sets Dr. Chinnaiyan's work apart from other books is the vital additional message that 'we are not our body-mind.' That is, while the wisdom of traditions such as Ayurveda do promote and sustain the health of the body-mind through diet and lifestyle, their ultimate value is the recognition of the primacy of consciousness and capacity to cultivate awareness beyond the body-mind of the Self, the true foundation of well-being."—Paul J. Mills, PhD, director and professor of family medicine and public health at UC San Diego's Center of Excellence for Research and Training in Integrative Health

"*The Heart of Wellness* details how the body can be an ally to self-inquiry, not an impediment. I recommend this unique book, whether your interest is physical health or spiritual enlightenment, or both."—Greg Goode, PhD, author of *After Awareness*, *The Direct Path*, and *Standing as Awareness*

"[This book] harnesses the power of our mind, senses, and spirit, the discovery of latent bliss, and admirably refutes our endless seeking of material things and desires."—Barry A. Franklin, PhD, FACSM, MAACVPR, FAHA, director of Preventive Cardiology and Cardiac Rehabilitation at William Beaumont Hospital

"Dr. Kavitha Chinnaiyan adeptly explains that bliss is created when you understand your true nature. With her cross-disciplinary expertise, Dr. Chinnaiyan guides you through diet, breathing exercises, and meditation, and helps you inhabit your body, mind, and spirit wholly and with true understanding...*The Heart of Wellness* is a compassionate guide offering a way for the totality of your being to experience true healing."—Pratima Raichur, author of *Absolute Beauty*

"In Dr. Chinnaiyan's passionate new book, she explores not only a modern approach to heart health through western medicine, diet, and exercise, but delves equally into the meaning of wellness and finding joy and bliss in health and disease."—Partha Nandi, MD, author of *Ask Dr. Nandi*

"*The Heart of Wellness* is an important read for health care professionals and their patients with the vision to look beyond the medical model."—Melvyn Rubenfire, MD, professor of internal medicine and director of preventive cardiology at the University of Michigan and editor of *Psychiatry and Heart Disease*

"*The Heart of Wellness* provides an intuitive, practical, and sensible approach to restoring balance and resilience. Kavitha has eloquently put together the Bliss Rx, taking the best from eastern philosophy and western science. I urge you to read this book."—Pankaj K. Vij, MD, author of *Turbo Metabolism* (New World Library, 2018)

"Dr. Kavitha Chinnaiyan has written a masterpiece...Readers will be emboldened and motivated to realize their true blissful nature."
—Todd C. Villines, MD, FACC, FAHA, FSCCT, professor of medicine at Uniformed Services University of the Health Science and director of cardiovascular research at Walter Reed National Military Medical Center

The
Heart of
Wellness

About the Author

Dr. Kavitha Chinnaiyan is a cardiologist and Professor of Medicine at Oakland University William Beaumont School of Medicine in Royal Oak, MI. She has studied Advaita Vedānta, Ayurveda, and Yoga with teachers across the globe. Her workshops, courses and writings on meditation, Yoga, Tantra, Ayurveda and non-duality strive to bring these time-honored traditions to modern living in practical ways. She is the author of *Shakti Rising* (Nonduality Press, October 2017), which won the Nautilus Gold Award for Best Books of 2017, and *Glorious Alchemy: Living the Lalitā Sahasranāma* (New Sarum Press, UK, January 2020). Visit her at kavithamd.com.

KAVITHA CHINNAIYAN, MD

The
Heart of
Wellness

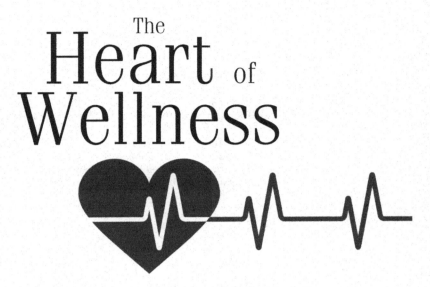

Transform Your Habits, Lifestyle, and Health

Sfaim Press

SECOND EDITION

Book design by Rebecca Zins
Cover design by Brianna Harden
Cover art by Rashmi Thirtha and Simi Jois
Illustrations on pages 108 and 218 by Mary Ann Zapalac

The information in this book is not meant to diagnose, treat, prescribe, or substitute consultation with a licensed healthcare professional. The author and the publisher assume no liability or responsibility for any complications that may arise as a result of the practices outlined in this book.

Publisher's Cataloging-In-Publication Data
(Prepared by The Donohue Group, Inc.)
Names: Chinnaiyan, Kavitha M., author.

Title: The heart of wellness : transform your habits, lifestyle, and health / Kavitha Chinnaiyan, MD.

Description: Second edition. | Northville, MI : Sfaim Press, [2020] | Includes bibliographical references and index.

Identifiers: ISBN 9781953023001 (paperback) | ISBN 9781953023018 (ePub) | ISBN 9781953023025 (mobi) | ISBN 9781953023032 (pdf)

Subjects: LCSH: Holistic medicine--Popular works. | Mind and body--Popular works. | Self-care, Health--Popular works.

Classification: LCC R733 .C487 2020 (print) | LCC R733 (ebook) | DDC 613--dc23

Any internet references contained in this work are current at publication time, but the publisher cannot guarantee that a specific location will continue to be maintained. Please refer to the publisher's website for links to authors' websites and other sources.

Sfaim Press
18999 Bella Vista Ct
Northville, MI 48168

Contents

Exercises

Foreword

Dr. Chinnaiyan offers an entirely new approach to "wellth" and illness. She calls the path Bliss Rx, which is a paradigm-expanding approach to health, illness, self, and peace that blends her strong roots in both Eastern tradition and practices and her cutting-edge practice of heart care at a major center. She asks the hard question, "What if we are more than just body and mind?" What if we have a pure light inside—one that radiates bliss, one that has been covered up and hidden by the twists and turns of life but that can be rediscovered to understand and deal with suffering?

I have had the joy of knowing Dr. Chinnaiyan for nearly two decades in my role as an attending cardiologist and teacher. Her potential for greatness was obvious. She raised lovely daughters, developed an excellence in the clinical practice of cardiology and research, and began to teach other trainees to grow to her level of a caring, intelligent, and effective clinician. Not many of us around were aware of the hours she was spending studying and practicing advanced yoga and meditation before and after working the long hours that her trade required.

We are fortunate that she persisted on these demanding paths because her introduction of her six-month program Heal Your Heart Free Your Soul stood out at this shrine of technology. Just a floor above her meetings were millions of dollars' worth of state-of-the-art CT and MRI scanners, ultrasound machines, and complex catheterization laboratories dedicated to exploring the workings and diseases that so commonly affect heart and arteries. At the same time, in her program on the first floor, hearts were being inspected with breath, silence, support, and calm.

Our good fortune is that Dr. Chinnaiyan has now distilled the profound experiences and gains she observed from her courses into a manual that challenges us to look within, slow down, and consider our lives. *The Heart of Wellness* is a paradigm shift in going beyond the body and mind that we are taught to consider in Western medicine (frankly, much more often the body than the mind). It brings an examination of spirituality and awakening from limitations that often are the root cause of pain and suffering of the heart and entire body.

Dr. Chinnaiyan doesn't promise us cures or disease reversal but uses her profound study of Ayurveda, Yoga, and Vedanta to present an opportunity to wake up to the blissfulness of our existence. This process may enhance healing as a side benefit, but it is worth pursuing on its own. This is not a seven-day or four-week radical cure but a life path that can be embraced at any pace at any time.

Although my path has not been as deeply steeped in Eastern traditions as that of my friend and now teacher Kavitha Chinnaiyan, it has included years of yoga and a period of practicing Kundalini yoga. The haunting music of that practice touched me deeply, as did the unusual flows that went on for an hour or more. Of the various chants I was exposed to, none touched me more than the words "I am the light of my soul, I am beautiful, I am bountiful, I am bliss, I am, I am." Dr. Chinnaiyan has written a primer to help us truly accomplish those words—to realize the bliss that is within and to use that bliss to address any health issues we may face. Once in a generation a book appears that defines a new paradigm in its field. *The Heart of Wellness* is that book for our generation. Your copy, like mine, will have corners bent over and pages highlighted to return to.

Joel K. Kahn, MD, FACC, clinical professor of medicine at
Wayne State University School of Medicine and author of
The Plant-Based Solution (Sounds True, 2018)

Acknowledgments

This book has been the amalgamation of the teachings of many who have graced my understanding of both life and medicine. I'm deeply grateful to the various teachers who sparked my interest in medicine as a young child and to those that gave it shape and momentum in medical school, residency, and cardiology fellowship. I'm fortunate to work with some of the best physicians in my field; they inspire me daily with their compassion, selflessness, and commitment to science and patient care.

I'm humbled to continue to learn from some of the finest teachers of Ayurveda, Yoga, and Vedanta—Swami Chinmayananda, whose writings on Vedanta fueled my fire of longing for truth; Yogani, the founder of Advanced Yoga Practices, who helped shape my understanding of Yoga; Greg Goode, whose teachings on the Direct Path shifted my perspective in a profound and permanent manner; Byron Katie, whose self-inquiry method has brought deeper understanding, joy, and peace to countless patients and participants of my program; Dr. Stuart Rothenberg and Dr. Nancy Lonsdorf of Maharishi Ayurveda, whose delightful and practical teaching of Ayurveda has made it easy for me to incorporate this great science in daily medical practice; and Dr. Sumit Kesarkar, whose teachings on Ayurveda, Yoga, and nondualism continue to shape my spiritual and medical practice. I'm grateful for the many teachers who shape my understanding through their work, books, papers, and talks. Thank you.

ACKNOWLEDGMENTS

My deep thanks go to Dr. Joel Kahn, my dear friend and colleague who guided me in the book-writing process, and to Lisa Hagan, my wonderful agent and friend for her uncompromising support and encouragement during this long and sometimes challenging writing process. I'm indebted to the wonderful team at Llewellyn for their advice that helped shape the format of this book. My special thanks to Angela Wix, my editor, for her insightful comments that helped clarify the message of the book.

Thank you to my wonderful friends who gave me valuable feedback as this book was taking shape, especially Drs. Beena Vesikar, Sarah D. Hashmi, Sridevi Gandrajpalli, Jaya Kumari, and Shylaja Swami. My deep thanks to David Kuttruff, whose feedback helped clarify my writing. Neither the Heal Your Heart program nor this book would have taken shape without the able and efficient help of my dear friend Ann DePetris. Thank you.

My heartfelt gratitude goes to all my patients who show me what medicine is really about. You give me more than I can ever give you—you help me grow as a human through your stories, frailty, courage, and grace. I'm humbled to interact with each of you.

I'm grateful to my parents, Nataraj and Geetha, whose selfless and unconditional love and support cannot be described in words. I love you. My loving thanks to my husband, Arul, who held space for me when I was juggling the roles of a full-time cardiologist, mother, wife, and writer. Thank you to my beautiful daughters, Anya and Annika, who continue to teach me the meaning of love and devotion.

Introduction

Kim sat across from me, anger and frustration etched on her face. "I can't believe this happened to me. I exercise every single day. I pay attention to every morsel that goes in my mouth. I don't smoke and have only two to three alcoholic drinks per year. All my five siblings are overweight; they all smoke and eat the unhealthiest foods. If anyone should get cancer, it should be one of them, not me."

I sat quietly, listening to her pain-filled words. She had just been diagnosed with breast cancer and was in my office for a preoperative cardiac evaluation. She began to sob softly. Why had good health eluded her even though she did everything right?

When her sobbing subsided, I gently asked her to tell me about her motivation to take such good care of herself. Frustration replaced the sadness in her voice as she described her parents' lifestyles—they both had been obese and had regularly binged on food, cigarettes, and alcohol before succumbing to heart disease in their sixties. She voiced her disappointment that her siblings had blindly followed the "doomed" path paved by their parents. I asked her if she felt that her siblings' choices made them more deserving of cancer. She began to cry again. "I can't believe I would want that for them, but I feel that they deserve it more than I do," she said quietly. I commended her for her honesty. Few of us would ever admit to having such thoughts! I asked her, "Who judges what each of us deserves?"

She remained quiet for several long moments before admitting that she didn't know. "If I do everything right, shouldn't it mean that I get to remain disease-free?" she asked.

"Well, you're sitting here with the diagnosis. What is the reality of the situation, whether or not it should have happened?" I asked.

She thought about it for a while and said, "The reality is that I'm here now."

"That's it. What should or should not happen and what should have or should not have happened are mere speculations. What if you never had the ability to think what should be?" I asked.

She sat quietly for a long time. "Then I'd still be sitting here, but without all this pain," she said with a smile.

Kim had touched upon the root cause of suffering, which is always separate from disease. After I'd examined her, I asked her to investigate her intentions for lifestyle changes and consider whether it came from a place of love for herself or fear of disease.

The Bliss Rx

How does it matter what the intention for wellness is and where it comes from? This is what we will explore in this book, which is not about curing heart disease. It is not even about preventing it with certainty. It is about healing the heart that beats tirelessly in the chest by revealing the heart that is the seat of our true nature.

Consider this question: Who are you? If you are like most of humanity, you might say you are so-and-so, with a particular name, ethnicity, culture, religion, political belief, and other stories that make up your life. You might define yourself by where and when you were born, the state of your body and mind, and your aspirations for the future. In other words, your identity is one of a body-mind occupying a particular time and space in the grand scheme of the universe.

How would your life be if you discovered that who you really are is eternal, unborn, and undying, and bliss is your essential nature? You might be tempted to throw this book away if this is not your current experience, but I implore you to read on. It is quite natural for us to believe that we are limited beings because that is the default model in which the world operates.

Starting at an early age, we are taught by well-meaning caregivers that we are fundamentally incomplete and limited, and that we must seek completion by "making something" of ourselves and "getting somewhere" in our lives. Our lives are marked by an endless seeking to overcome the overpowering sense of lack that arises from believing ourselves to be limited and flawed. We seek happiness from the outside in the form of wealth, fame, achievement, success, love, security, and relationships.

As we will see in this book, suffering is the result of taking ourselves to be the body-mind. As long as this identity remains, we will suffer because we will always seek completion from external objects. No matter how much we seek and for how long, lasting happiness evades us. We will never have only joy, success, health, and the other things that are desirable. We come to see that life is a zero-sum game—we get what we want some of the time and what we don't want at other times. Our life is marked by chasing what we want and avoiding what we don't want. Since the outcome of anything we do is never in our hands, we live with an underlying sense of uncertainty, dissatisfaction, and yearning, and we never experience lasting contentment.

In contrast to the default model, the bliss model is based on the principle that who we are is much more than the body-mind. Our true nature is pure bliss consciousness: we are unborn and undying, and the body-mind is a mere reflection of our eternal nature. When we realize this, we develop a deep reverence and gratitude for the gift of embodiment, and suffering drops away. There is nothing we can seek outside of ourselves because we see that we are already whole. When bliss permeates our senses, minds, bodies, thoughts, and emotions, our relationship with ourselves, disease, others, and the world changes to one of absolute beauty and joy. Merely believing that we are bliss is not enough; we have to know it experientially. Only then can its transformative power heal us. For this knowing to occur, the various layers of misconceptions about who we think we are must be peeled away. This is the goal of the Bliss Rx.

The Origins of the Bliss Rx

The principles and practices described in this book represent a fundamental shift in our understanding of who we are; they are about healing and are not necessarily a cure. With a shift in the model through which we operate, we can heal completely without being cured of disease. This approach is far removed from the principles of modern medicine, where we become fixated on getting rid of disease at all costs. I am often asked how all this came about. How is it that a cardiologist trained in Western medicine is called to prescribe bliss?

Many parts of this story may seem familiar to you. I had been studying Yoga for several years when I was attracted to a career in medicine. The busy coursework of medical school drew me in, and Yoga moved to the back burner. Competitive and ambitious, I progressed through medical school, internal medicine residency, and cardiology fellowship, getting married and having a family amidst the rigors of training. Midway through residency I became aware of a nagging sense of dissatisfaction that poked its head up quite often; there was always something more to achieve. I wondered why no achievement or success brought lasting peace. However, this ennui seemed to be normal; everyone I knew was also seeking something more.

This inner conflict reached a fever pitch at the start of my training in cardiology. I had just given birth to my second child and couldn't be happier—yet even the beauty and purity of motherhood hadn't permanently erased the sense of inner dissatisfaction. Now I worried about balancing my work with my family and how to progress in my career without losing touch with my children. At each stage of life a new ambition had replaced the old one, and the seeking continued.

One Saturday morning I was unloading the dishwasher when my eyes rested briefly on the block of kitchen knives. I wondered casually if death could end this inner conflict. The thought arose from curiosity; I wasn't depressed or suicidal. Quite suddenly the thought gave way to a vivid vision. I saw myself as a deeply unfulfilled old woman exhausted from the endless cascade of seeking; the permanent contentment that I sought had eluded me despite a successful career and family life. The feeling wasn't one of greed or of wanting more but that of utter despair that I had missed the most important lesson in life.

As the vision faded and my awareness returned to the kitchen, I noticed that several minutes had passed and my hand was frozen in mid-air, still clutching a utensil. I sat down, shaking. Finally, I knew that what I was really seeking was the end of seeking. No amount of gathering, achieving, or acquiring anything from the external world would solve this puzzle. The quest for the key to this puzzle took me on the inner journey that would lead to a paradigm shift.

Finishing up my cardiology training, I began my clinical practice, waking up well before dawn and spending hours in meditation and self-inquiry before my children rose and the day began. After I put them to bed at night, I read voraciously and meditated again. Guided by many teachers along the way, I learned to question all that I had taken to be true—my beliefs, thoughts, emotions, actions, and life itself. My life began to change gradually, and this transformation exuded outward in an expanding circle to include family, friends, and patients. This journey had opened the doors to vast possibilities and realms I had never imagined. The model through which I operated began to shift.

Patients were no longer body-minds that needed "fixing" but were vibrant expressions of bliss that were inseparable from me. How could I keep talking about their disease as if they were their disease? How could I prescribe medicines, procedures, or surgeries and send them on their way without trying to have them see their own inherent perfection? How could I possibly have them believe that fixing their disease was the way to end their suffering or that incurable disease meant endless suffering? I was ridden with conflict between my own self-discovery and the way I was practicing medicine. It felt incomplete and phony to not address the elements that contributed to both disease and healing—the mental, psychological, social, emotional, and economic issues that make up our identities and stories. It was not enough to ask people to eat right, start exercising, and stop smoking without also asking them to examine the stress and tensions of reacting and responding to life in fixed, conditioned ways. And yet, I had no reference for how to address these issues from my training in modern medicine. I turned to Ayurveda, Yoga, and Vedanta for answers.

Ayurveda

Ayurveda, literally translated as "knowledge of life," is one of the oldest medical systems, having originated nearly 5,000 years ago. It is a comprehensive science with a philosophy that everything in creation is interconnected; therefore, the health of our body is deeply related to our mind, senses, spirit, and the world we live in. As I began to study Ayurveda, a series of light bulbs began to switch on in my understanding of life, health, and disease. The many gaps of modern medicine that were evident in my training were gradually filled up.

I continue to study the science with various teachers across the globe. My own practice of Yoga has been deeply enriched by incorporating Ayurvedic principles; this came as no surprise since Yoga and Ayurveda are sister sciences.

Yoga

The word Yoga is derived from the root *yuj* ("to join") and can refer to the joining of many things: breath with body, breath with awareness, individual with God, skillful action, dispassion and nonattachment to one's lower self (the limited body-mind), unity with the higher self (eternal bliss consciousness), and so on. Mostly, however, Yoga is defined as the discovery of our true nature of bliss, which occurs when all our mental modifications come to rest.

In Yoga we are asked to cultivate positive aspects of our bodies and minds by discriminating between what serves us and what doesn't. By constantly redirecting our focus and attention, we stop trying to find happiness in external objects. With this, our mental modifications and discursive mind activity come to a rest and we realize that who we are is eternal bliss consciousness. With this shift in identity and perspective, health and disease take on a very different meaning. We find that many of our ailments seem to disappear, and those that don't no longer bind us in suffering.

The eightfold path of Yoga consists of the following limbs: moral or ethical injunctions (nonviolence, truth, non-stealing, celibacy, and non-clinging), virtues (purity, contentment, perseverance, self-reflection, and devotion), body postures, regulation of breath (known as pranayama), withdrawal of senses, one-pointed contemplation, meditation, and absorption into the object of meditation. Self-inquiry is an additional practice that comes from Vedanta.

Vedanta

Vedanta is a secular science that translates into "end of knowledge." It looks critically into our existence and the source of suffering. The end of knowledge here refers to the end of seeking external objects for our happiness or to feel complete—material objects like wealth or nonmaterial objects like fame, success, love, sense pleasures, or relationships. As I discovered years ago, such seeking never ends because one thing leads to another in an endless loop of desires. Vedanta teaches us to look at our life, our body, and our mind in a highly logical fashion. By contemplating existential questions, we come to see that what we are cannot be separate from what we know.

Ordinarily, when we talk about knowledge, we are referring to knowledge about something—I go to medical school to learn about health and disease. When I become a doctor, I know about medicine; I don't become it. Yet, when I call myself a doctor, my knowledge about medicine becomes who I think I am. We identify with our knowledge about things—a lawyer knows about law, a botanist knows about plants, a herpetologist knows about snakes. This is known as secular knowledge. Our entire education system is based on secular knowledge, which also forms the basis of our experience.

When we look deeply into the experience of sense objects, we will see that we refer to knowledge about seeing or hearing when we look at an object or hear a sound. When we say "I see," we are really saying that we know that seeing is happening. Without the knowing or the aware-ness of seeing, we wouldn't be able to see. When we say "I see a bird," we are referring to the knowledge about the bird gained through seeing. Throughout our waking hours, we accumulate knowledge about the world through our senses or about our inner landscape by being aware of thoughts and emotions. Secular knowledge becomes the basis of our experience and identity. For example, if a stressful situation comes along, I become identified with it as "I am stressed," when in fact it is only an experience. Vedanta teaches us to examine knowledge critically: if knowl-edge of my experience is not who I am, then who am I?

This inquiry leads us to Self-knowledge, or knowledge about our true nature. The capital "S" differentiates it from the self with the small "s" that we think we are—the body-mind. The body and the mind, along with the countless experiences that become our identity, are objects, while the Self is the sole subject. Objects are temporary, while the subject is per-manent, unchanging, ever-blissful. Knowledge of our true blissful nature puts an end to becoming identified with objects of experience.

Practicing the Bliss Rx

As my self-discovery progressed, I began teaching select patients to med-itate during their clinic visits. Initially, they were mainly patients with heavy symptom loads of palpitations, chest pain, shortness of breath, and other complaints. Among the patients that kept up the practice, the results were astounding: they would return with significantly decreased symptoms. Some patients were no longer interested in meditation for reducing symptoms but for the other benefits it provided, such as peace, a sense of calm amidst activity, better sleep and mood, and a changing outlook toward life. They began to request classes they could attend and recommend to their loved ones, which led to the Heal Your Heart Free Your Soul program.

For six months, from October to March, we met at the department auditorium where I taught various practices, beginning with meditation and progressing to additional practices such as breathing techniques and self-inquiry. The program ended with a weekend retreat of intense practices. At the end of the first six-month session, there was a waiting list of people who had heard about the program. When we examined the benefits of the program, we found a significant improvement among participants in measures of perceived stress and mental and emotional components of health over the six-month period.[1]

Although the program initially included people with heart disease, it began to attract those with other chronic ailments such as cancer. Soon, people with no disease or issues started enrolling in the program to discover a holistic way to be happy, healthy, and fulfilled.

Can Self-Discovery Be Measured?

Progress on the path of self-discovery is mostly subjective. Although there are sophisticated ways of measuring brain activity to infer one's mental state, the resting of the mind to reveal our true nature is largely unquantifiable. How we respond to life and to our own minds changes and becomes filled with sweetness, softness, and acceptance—parameters that are difficult to measure objectively. Physiological responses such as heart rate, blood pressure, and hormone and biomarker levels or healthcare outcomes such as the need for medications and procedures, hospital admissions, symptom relief, quality of life, and changes in lifestyle may or may not correlate with nonmeasurable parameters such as perception and outlook on life.

This is a significant challenge in body-mind research since subjective improvements surpass objective measurements that the scientific community thrives on. Many studies have demonstrated the beneficial effects of Yoga, meditation, mindfulness, and other body-mind approaches on heart disease and other chronic illnesses. In this book there will be little emphasis on objective measures. Instead, the approach here is on the subtle aspects of this path on our relationship with ourselves (including our health and illnesses) and with the world.

---

1   K. M. Chinnaiyan, A. M. DePetris, J. A. Boura, K. Stakich-Alpirez, and S. S. Billecke, "Feasibility of Establishing a Comprehensive Yoga Program and Its Dose-Effect Relationship on Cardiovascular Risk Factors and Wellness Parameters: A Pilot Study," *Int J Yoga Therap* 25 (2015): 135–40.

Building Blocks of the Bliss Rx

The program outlined in this book is based on the following principles:

Model: This program is not aimed toward curing or preventing heart disease; rather, its goal is to optimize the working of the body-mind so that the bliss of our true nature can be revealed. In the process of optimization disease and stress may be reversed, but this is not the end goal.

Science: Many scientific disciplines are interwoven in this book, including neuroscience, physiology, psychology, and quantum physics. Whenever available, modern theories are presented side by side with those of Ayurveda, Yoga, and Vedanta to understand the similarities and differences between them.

Holistic: Every aspect of the program fits into all the other aspects, like a jigsaw puzzle. All the practices complement each other; the whole is greater than the sum of its parts.

Logic: Practices of the program are based on sound logic and are therefore secular and not based in any faith or religion. People who have followed this program have found it to be complementary to their religious beliefs.

Timeless: The strength of a comprehensive program like this one is that you never lose what you gain. Even if you pick it up years after dropping it, you will make progress.

Pace: This program is meant to be self-paced. There is no set time limit for each step, and you can take as long as you need.

Simplicity: The program is simple; however, simple doesn't mean easy. It will ask you to change your fundamental thinking about yourself, others, and the world. It is not meant to be a bandage or cover-up of deeper issues but a radical shift in your perspective that will lead you from suffering to bliss.

How to Use This Book

This book is laid out in two parts. Part 1 begins with the fundamental difference between the default and the bliss models. Here we will examine the scientific literature and evidence for the program, the logic behind it, and why such an approach is meaningful. We will examine the differences between the two models when it comes to heart disease and its risk factors and the heart-mind connection. We will understand the true meaning of a holistic approach, which neither negates modern medicine nor elevates ancient wisdom but integrates both. Part 2 consists of the Bliss Rx, with distinct steps for realizing bliss as our true nature.

There is no single way to read and implement the recommendations laid out in this book. Here are some suggestions:

- You can read from beginning to end, as with any other book. Feel free to include the exercises or skip them initially. Once you've read through, return to part 2 and do the exercises as recommended.

- If part 1 is too onerous or dense, skip it and go directly to part 2. Alternatively, read the chapter summaries of part 1 and move on to part 2. If you are curious about the science behind the particular aspects of the program, then you can read the relevant sections or chapters in part 1.

- I recommend keeping a journal to record your inner and outer progress. Write down your experiences, insights, and discoveries as you progress through the program.

Disclaimer

While on this program, it is important to continue with the medicines prescribed by your doctor. You may find that your need for medicines may decline. At every visit with your doctor, ask about your medicines, what they are for, and how your need for them can be evaluated (through blood tests, drug holidays, and so on). This approach is not meant to conflict with your current regimen; it is meant to be complementary.

This is not a book on Ayurvedic medicine or self-healing. We will not go into body typing and laying out specific guidelines based on quizzes (though in the resources section I've listed some excellent books that are based on Ayurvedic body typing). Instead, it uses the guiding principles of Ayurveda, Yoga, and Vedanta to address the root cause of suffering. The approach taken here regarding health and wellness is that a healthy body-mind makes it easier for us to let go of the mental modifications that obscure our true blissful nature. The whole purpose of the program is to enable this great self-discovery, not for mere healing of the body-mind. Along the way, such healing can (and often does) occur, but that is only a side benefit and not the end point.

Exercise: Clarifying Intention

As we discovered in Kim's story, our intention for change forms the basis for our actions and what comes of our actions. The outcome of our actions always reflects our intention, which can often be unclear or hidden. To make progress in any field, we must know what we want before we go about taking action. For example, in smoking cessation programs, setting a quit date is the most important first step. If I set the intention but don't really want to quit smoking, the program will not work for me.

Similarly, if you don't really want to discover the unlimited bliss of who you are, you will not feel like keeping up with the program when your mind stories and life situations pull you back into suffering. The drama of the body-mind will seem far more alluring.

- Before you begin practicing the techniques in part 2, take time to think about what you really want. Write down your answer on a small piece of paper, keeping it limited to one sentence.

- Once you are satisfied with your answer, fold the paper and keep it in your wallet. It can be as simple as "I want to realize lasting joy and peace that can manifest as health and wellness" or "I want my combative relationship with my disease to come to an end" or "I want to understand why I'm not always happy and discover ways to find lasting joy."

- Now that you know what you want, set an intention to realize your desire. Hold it close in your heart and think about it as you go about your day. Take out the note and read it, particularly when you feel unmotivated to follow through.

Setting intentions works wonders in every area of life. I make a ritual out of it in order to infuse it with sincerity and longing. It can be a simple thing like being present for my children on the weekend. Every time I'm distracted, I remember the intention I made that is infused with the love I have for them and the awareness of how fleeting their childhood is. Immediately my attitude, posture, and attention shift into one of being completely immersed in what they are saying or doing. Everything else can wait because now is the time for me to honor my intention to myself, and in this honoring, my children benefit as much as I do.

The beauty of this path is that even if you are half-hearted about it, sticking with it will transform your desire and intention. As you progress through the Bliss Rx, you will gain greater clarity and insight into your deepest desires and longings.

The only other ingredient required for this program is integrity, which is honesty in action. Small steps taken with integrity and commitment are much more effective than ambitious plans that we can't really keep up with. At all times, recall that the path to bliss is your birthright. There is nobody that is more or less deserving of it, for it is the true nature of all in existence. Mostly, enjoy the process!

In the next chapter we will explore the many benefits of the Bliss Rx and the ways in which this program transforms our life, health, and relationship with disease.

Summary

- The principles and practices described in this book represent a fundamental paradigm shift in our understanding of who we are, which determines our relationship with health and disease.

- In the default model we assume that we are the body, the mind, or a combination of the two. This model leads to endless seeking because it is associated with an inherent sense of lack, so we continually seek fulfillment from external objects.

- In the bliss model we start with the knowledge that who we are is eternal bliss consciousness. When we see this, we stop seeking for completion because we realize that we are already blissfully whole. This realization changes our relationship with ourselves, the world, and our disease. Suffering drops away.

- The approach taken in this book is that a healthy body-mind makes it easier for us to realize our true blissful nature. The whole purpose of the program is to enable this great self-discovery and not for mere healing of the body-mind.

- Before you begin the program, clarify your desire and set an intention to work with it.

Part 1

Models of Health and Disease

In this section we will investigate the fundamental differences between the default and the bliss models, including scientific literature and evidence for both. We will delve into the limitations of the default model and study the logic behind the bliss model and how such an approach can be practical, useful, and meaningful. Importantly, we will see that a truly holistic approach negates neither model but harmoniously incorporates both. We will begin with the end in mind by assessing the manifold benefits of such an integrative model.

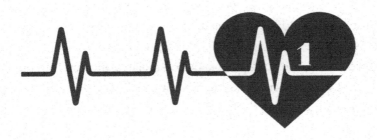

Healing in the
Bliss Rx Program

The Bliss Rx is targeted toward discovering bliss. In this program you will work in an outside-in fashion to clear out everything that obscures bliss; by doing so, you will bring every aspect of your life back into balance.

When bliss begins to permeate our senses, our minds, our hearts, and our actions, health is restored in an inside-out fashion. Does this mean that blockages in arteries and leaky valves will be miraculously cured? Maybe. Maybe not. But what this means is that with the end of suffering, these conditions will not limit us in any way. They will become irrelevant as they are gently accepted into our reality. Once the bliss of our true nature is tasted, nothing else will seem as sweet or as worthy of our attention and devotion. When we begin to live our lives as bliss, we change the structure of the cosmos. Yes, each of us is that significant and that powerful.

Every choice, every thought, and every action that occurs daily takes us one step toward or away from bliss—and, by default, health. Nothing can be excluded in our pursuit of bliss: the way we brush our teeth, greet our spouse, look in the mirror, talk to the waitress, drive our car, prepare our food, eat our meals, exercise our body, nurture our mind, and relate to our children, colleagues, customers, or parents. Everything counts. It is not just what we do but how we do it that makes a world of difference in whether we are moving closer to suffering or to bliss.

Once we tap into it, bliss expands and radiates outward into our body, mind, and world, permeating them with its joyful and peaceful essence. The following are some of the effects of this inside-out process.

Reduced Stress

If you follow the practices of this program, my hope is that you will experience a greater sense of calmness and an ability to deal with the stressors you face in daily life. The meditation practice alone will have the effect of decreasing the stress response.

Shift in Stimulus for Lifestyle Changes

When it comes to the effectiveness of the program on health and disease, perhaps the most dramatic shift we can see is in why we make lifestyle changes. In the default model, lifestyle changes are made out of fear and resistance—we change how we eat, we start exercising, and we quit unhealthy addictions because we worry about getting a disease or dying before our time. The fear of disease or death hangs constantly like a sword over our heads, the ominous voice commenting on every choice we make.

In the bliss model, lifestyle changes occur out of a deep honoring of our bodies and minds. The wonder of being alive arises not only as a joyful respect for the body's miraculous processes but also aligns us with all of life. We intuitively reach for foods, exercise, and entertainment that honors this inherent joy. While our progress in the program occurred in an outside-in fashion, it now proceeds in an inside-out fashion, our choices radiating from the wellspring of inner bliss.

Loss of Victimization

When we delve into self-inquiry practices, we realize that the stories we have been telling ourselves have no inherent truth. When we cultivate the ability to stand apart from our stories, we see that believing these stories placed us in the role of victim. When we take responsibility for our own mental processes and actions, we stop reacting and start responding. With this responsibility, we stop being victims and grow into self-mastery.

We realize that no other person, history, situation, or circumstance is responsible for the way we think, act, and feel. When we take back the power for our thoughts, feelings, and actions, we learn to stand in the light of our own bliss. We lose the ability to ask "Why me?" or "What did I do to deserve this?"

Discovery of Forgiveness

When we stop being victims of our circumstances, situations, or others, we become radically forgiving. The concept of forgiveness shifts and we realize that in the spaciousness of the here and now, neither the past nor the future exist as reality. We see that our grudges and hang-ups take away power from ourselves and place it upon our situations and others. We see that we don't forgive for others' sake. It is a natural outcome of loss of suffering. Moreover, when we reclaim our power, we see that forgiveness is not something we do. It is what happens when we stop being victims of our pasts, situations, and others.

Discovery of Compassion

Compassion is the natural consequence of loss of victimization and discovery of forgiveness. Note that compassion is different from pity, which has the connotation of superiority. We pity someone that we think is beneath us.

Compassion, on the other hand, is rooted in love and equality. When I see that I'm as much of a slave to my conditioning as everyone else, I stop judging them. I see that the only reason I'm bothered about something in you is that I have the same trait. Empathy replaces judgment and wholeness replaces separateness. My understanding of your predicament is not based in thoughts about how things should be for you, which would be arrogant. How can I possibly know what should or should not be? Instead, I open fully to your pain and allow it to be. You and I become one in the spaciousness of being. Your pain is honored in this openness and availability. All possibilities are held in love.

Discovery of Gratitude

When the grip of conditioning is loosened, we lose the ordinary way of living in the head and move into the spaciousness of the body. In this spaciousness we begin to engage with the world in a novel way. Sense perceptions, physical sensations, thoughts, and emotions become vibrant and alive. With the shift of our mental processes we tend to live in the moment. With this transition to openness we discover an inherent sweetness in all of life. Wishing for something other than what is stops making sense. Wanting a specific outcome also stops making sense. The wonder of being takes over even though life goes on as before, and there is immense gratitude for it. The flavor of our prayer changes from one of needing and wanting to one of overwhelming gratitude for the gift of life.

Growing Acceptance

When we discover the vast, empty spaciousness within, our relationship with life, health, and disease takes a dramatic turn. Nothing is the enemy. If you have a chronic illness, you will start to notice a deep gratitude towards it. It becomes the doorway for self-discovery and you put your weapons down. Your attitude toward treatment will change; of course you will pursue the best therapies for your condition, take your medications, and follow your doctor's orders, but the why of it shifts.

While in the past treatment was based on fear and rejection ("I don't want to have it," "I don't want to die," "I want my old life back," and so on), it is now based in growing acceptance. Thoughts and concepts about disease no longer make sense when you become adept at allowing sensations to arise and subside. You see that all fearful thoughts about wanting or not wanting and should or should not are arisings in the now. They have no inherent truth, and you can no longer take them seriously. This is true surrender.

Note: Many who have experienced a spontaneous cure or a remission attribute it to this deep acceptance. However, the paradox is this: it doesn't happen as long as your intention for acceptance is a cure or a remission. Only when you let go of wanting and totally allow everything to be as it is can the body heal to such a large extent.

The effects of the Bliss Rx described above will become a reality for you once you start applying the practices and principles that are presented in part 2. We will now examine the scientific basis for the default and bliss models. If you can't wait to get started, you can skip over to part 2 and return to the related sections as you read and practice.

Summary

- The Bliss Rx is targeted toward discovering bliss. In this program you will work in an outside-in fashion to bring every aspect of your life back into balance.

- Balance enables us to recognize our innate blissful perfection. When bliss begins to permeate our senses, our minds, our hearts, and our actions, health is restored and radiates outward in an inside-out fashion.

- Stress reduction is the most obvious first effect of the Bliss Rx.

- In the bliss model, lifestyle changes occur out of a deep honoring of our bodies and minds.

- When we take responsibility for our own mental processes and actions, we stop reacting and start responding, thereby growing into self-mastery and losing the victim mentality.

- When we reclaim our power and stop being victims, forgiveness arises naturally.

- Compassion is the natural consequence of loss of victimization and discovery of forgiveness.

- When we open to life in sweetness, we learn the meaning of acceptance. The wonder of being alive takes over and immense gratitude begins to arise.

- Naturally, our relationship with life, health, and disease takes a dramatic turn. If you have a chronic illness, you will start to notice a deep gratitude towards it. It becomes the doorway for self-discovery.

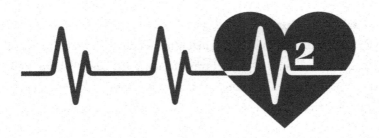

The Default and
the Bliss Models

Cindy was fifty-two when she first came to see me for her symptoms. Superbly articulate, intelligent, and curious, she eloquently described her condition. She had been having a constellation of symptoms for about two years and had undergone a battery of tests that didn't show any problems with her heart. Because she had a strong family history of heart disease, she was concerned even though the tests were negative.

When we talked about her life, she said that although she had a postgraduate degree, she had chosen to stay home to care for her children. Her voice was tinged with warmth and pride as she told me how well they were doing as young adults. She had gone back to work two years ago, plunging into the rat race. Her work was extremely stressful and she often stayed up late to finish projects. She had no time to cook, exercise, or relax, even on weekends. Her work consumed her. She had developed sciatica and arthritis, which made it difficult to exercise even when she had the time. She frequently suffered severe heartburn, palpitations, and chest pain. Her blood pressure and cholesterol were very high, and she admitted that she hated taking medications.

When she finished talking, we sat in silence for a few moments. I asked her to take a minute to tell me why she was working. She thought about it for a while and answered that she didn't need the money. She was doing it to feel the satisfaction of accomplishment. She said that she had been reading about her health problems and was "trying" to make changes but couldn't do what needed to be done. She was stunned when I told her that her body simply doesn't care how she felt about her work, her sense of accomplishment, or how hard she was trying.

Your Body Doesn't Care

As you will see in the following chapters, your body merely responds to the hormonal and chemical onslaughts brought on by particular pathways in the brain. Your arteries, organs, and cells simply don't have the ability to concern themselves with how hard you are trying to change your diet, develop an exercise habit, or cope with your life. They merely respond to what you do and how you think and feel. Your organs only see the end product of your effort and have no ability to appreciate the process. They don't care that you work hard to support your family, that you need success to feel good about yourself, or how much you hate your disease. How you feel about the world, politics, religion, other people, or yourself makes no difference to your body. Your financial and relationship issues, experiences of your past, and dreams for your future don't concern it either.

Your body takes in the energy it needs and expends just enough of it to keep the cells working. Your habits and addictions have a direct effect on your body through the brain and the hormonal system. If you're at war with the world or with yourself, your body notices and produces the hormones and chemicals that prepare you for fighting. If you're at peace, it reflects accordingly. It's not personal; it's biological.

As we spoke, I noticed a change in Cindy's posture. Her face lit up with recognition, and she exclaimed that she got it. She understood that her body was simply responding to her stressful lifestyle and resolved to change her situation immediately. She was receptive to the many changes

I suggested in her lifestyle, most of which are presented in this book. Over the next year I saw a considerable change in her attitude. She quit her job for a more relaxed consulting gig. She made time to rewire her brain, and her body responded accordingly. Her blood pressure came down and her heartburn went away. As her hormones began to return to a more wholesome balance, her cholesterol started decreasing without medications.

Why would Cindy's symptoms improve with a change in her attitude and, consequently, her lifestyle? After all, she was living the life that most of us can only dream of: a fulfilling (albeit stressful) job, successful parenting and marriage, and generally what we would consider a well-lived life. Isn't this what each of us strives for? Isn't this what we value? We appreciate success at any cost, even though the definition of success is fluid and subjective. Cindy's many symptoms related to her lifestyle form the basis of the model on which modern society operates. At the crux of this model lies the issue of identification.

The Default Model

In modern medicine the body forms the model for our identity. We assume that the body is who we really are. It is the basis for every aspect of our lives—from the way we live to what we seek to be happy to how we interact with others, form habits and lifestyle choices, and think about disease and death. In recent decades research on the effect of emotions and the mind on health has opened us to broadening our model a bit further—we may not think we are exclusively the body, but we feel that we are the body and the mind. When we operate from this assumption, we understand that the body isn't the entity that feels, makes decisions and choices, relates in relationships, or responds to the environment; rather, it is the mind, which is a large, amorphous mish-mash of thoughts and emotions. When the mind goes to the extremes of anxiety, depression, hallucinations, or psychosis, we tend to call it abnormal. Otherwise, we assume that the way we think, feel, and respond is normal because we see that everybody around us is behaving in the same way.

When we take ourselves to be our stories, we strive to avoid suffering at all costs, which may lead us to doggedly pursue diet, exercise, and lifestyle interventions in fanatical ways. The explosion of "cure-all therapies" in the current landscape of healthcare is proof of the default model—doctors and healthcare practitioners in all fields have seemingly come up with the ultimate diet, supplement, or lifestyle that is supposed to cure everything from heart disease to cancer. It isn't uncommon for me to see patients who jump from one such "cure" to another (and spend considerable amounts of money and resources in the effort) for years before concluding that none of these cures live up to their claims. They are looking to end suffering, yes, but they are looking in the wrong place.

Likes and Dislikes: The Fuel for Identity

When we identify ourselves as the body-mind, we are naturally driven to pursue what we like or what we think is good and avoid what we dislike or what we think is bad. We live our lives seeking pleasure and fulfillment in material and mental objects. Material objects are those that we can buy with money, whereas mental objects are those that we seek to feel complete: fame, notoriety, success, love, relationships, athletic achievements, and so on. Powered by certain brain and hormonal pathways, this endless seeking pervades all spheres of life, and we attribute our happiness or unhappiness to what we get or don't get.

We try to hold on to the good things, but they never last—the newer car model becomes more attractive than the one we have, fame comes and goes, spouses die, and children grow up. Even if the good things do last, they don't seem to give us the same extent of joy that they initially did. After thirty years in the same job, we feel uninspired and long for more. After a while, the big house we saved up for feels burdensome with all the maintenance. We go on diets, pursue extensive exercise programs, and invest in anti-aging products, finding that the body ages despite our best efforts.

When we don't have the things we want, we crave them. When we get what we want, we fear losing them. Our default "pull and push" mode of operation determines the way we relate to ourselves and others. Constant evaluation, judgment, and comparison form the basis of relationships—we like some people and dislike others. This attitude would be fine if we always get what we want and never what we don't want, but because life doesn't work that way, we have a constant underlying sense of being powerless. Our likes and dislikes become the labels that form our identity; they become who we are.

Having an incurable ailment like heart disease in this situation is devastating. Since we don't like having chronic diseases, our dislike of disease becomes our source of suffering. We want to do away with the disease because it threatens our identity. Prevention and treatment in this default model are thus based on the assumption that having what we want determines our happiness or suffering. Disease becomes the enemy that needs to be destroyed, as we see with the widespread "fights against" cancer, heart, or Alzheimer's disease.

Are Disease and Suffering Interchangeable?

The default model is also the basis for training in modern medicine. We are taught to focus entirely on the disease and very little on the person. The fundamental belief of operating in this model is that suffering is caused by disease. Everything we do to alleviate suffering stems from striving to make the disease go away. However, here is a sobering fact: very few diseases that afflict wealthy and developed nations are curable. Most of the illnesses we see in western medical practice are never cured—at most, they are "managed."

For example, congestive heart failure is the number-one cause for hospital admissions and readmissions in the US.[2] There is no cure for heart failure. The most definitive treatment for heart failure is heart transplantation or the newly approved ventricular-assist devices that take over the pumping function of the heart. The body's immune response never accepts the organ as its own and aggressively rejects it. Heavy-duty drugs

2   A. S. Go, D. Mozaffarian, and V. L. Roger, et al., "Heart disease and stroke statistics—2014 update: a report from the American Heart Association," *Circulation* 129 (2014): e28–e292.

that are given to overcome this immune reaction come with risks of common and rare infections, blood clots, and other fatal side effects. Nearly every transplanted heart develops a peculiar type of blockage in the coronary arteries that can cause heart attacks and death. We just replace one problem with another—even though we replace a diseased heart, suffering never ends even as quality of life is improved and people with transplanted hearts live longer than those who can't get one.

This predicament is not unique to heart failure; it is the case with every chronic illness that has no cure. As a nation, we spend billions of dollars in merely managing chronic incurable illnesses, which then begs the following question: Since the default model rests on the assumption that to end suffering we must make a disease go away, are we doomed to suffer if we can't get rid of disease? Conversely, does suffering go away if a disease is cured? Look at anyone who has been cured of a disease to see if they find lasting happiness. You'll find that they have something else that keeps them from realizing permanent happiness.

My training and practice in India took place among the very impoverished who had little access to healthcare. Infectious diseases like cholera, typhoid, and malaria predominated the hospital wards I worked in; there was much suffering among patients and their loved ones. The constant threat of death loomed large in communities subjected to not-too-rare outbreaks of water- and food-borne illnesses. It made sense, then, that disease would indeed cause suffering, and ending them should bring permanent happiness. However, this was not the case. Once cured of their disease, they continued to suffer because their attention shifted to other things they wanted and didn't have.

When I moved to America, it took me a while to become accustomed to practicing medicine differently. There has been no threat of imminent death from malaria or typhoid in the hospitals where I've worked. For the most part, doctors here deal with preventing chronic illnesses or their effects on quality of life. And yet there is no dearth of suffering even in this wealthy and privileged society. I learned that imagined outcomes of disease are as threatening to one's well-being as actual ones. For instance, anxiety about not recovering and fear of dying leads to worse outcomes in people who have had a heart attack.[3, 4] If we aren't battling disease, we are battling the world, others, and our own minds to find fulfillment.

Over the years of talking with hundreds of patients, I have come to see that suffering has nothing to do with disease and everything to do with the default model of taking our bodies to be who we are. As long as disease is the enemy, it is bound to cause suffering, no matter where we live and what our societal status is, and being cured of disease doesn't necessarily alleviate suffering as long as we operate from the default model.

The Bliss Model

Consider a statement like this, which is common in hospital charts: "John had been in good health until recently, when he was diagnosed with lung cancer." Our definition of John's health is that he didn't have cancer or any other known illness until recently. Notice that the definition doesn't say anything about his mind, emotions, or life. He could have had chronic stress and his life might have been in shambles, but the statement about his health doesn't really take into account anything but the absence of disease. This is in direct contradiction to the definition of health by the World Health Organization, which states that health is "a state of complete physical, mental, and social well-being and not merely the absence of disease or infirmity."

Ayurveda takes it one step further, stating that health is a state of perfect balance in which all bodily functions are normal, including digestion, tissue metabolism, and excretion. In health the mind, senses, and the self are filled with bliss.

The word *bliss* never came up in my medical training. In the default model we don't aim for bliss, particularly when there are no objective measures for it. There are no randomized controlled trials that look at

---

3   P. J. Tully, H. R. Winefield, and R. A. Baker, et al., "Depression, anxiety, and major adverse cardiovascular and cerebrovascular events in patients following coronary artery bypass graft surgery: a five-year longitudinal cohort study," *Biopsychosoc Med 9* (2015): 14.

4   A. Steptoe, G. J. Molloy, and N. Messerli-Bürgy, et al., "Fear of dying and inflammation following acute coronary syndrome," *Eur Heart J 32* (2011): 2405–11.

bliss as an end point. Instead, we focus on measurable end points such as procedures, deaths, heart attacks, or drug side effects. Notice that all these end points are squarely based on the default model that says we are the body-minds subject to disease and death.

Assumptions About the Brain

The default model is based on the assumption that the brain creates consciousness. However, we will see in the following chapters that the brain can only create electrical and hormonal pathways based on how we view life. It doesn't create consciousness that then powers the rest of the body-mind, since it is itself a part of the body.

Like the rest of the body-mind, the brain is subject to the same intelligence that powers our cells, organs, and tissues, which "know" exactly what they need to do—and don't need our direction or supervision, thank goodness! Imagine trying to make sure that your digestive system is breaking down that pizza, beer, and cake you had last night while orchestrating your heartbeat, immune system, and the countless chemical reactions that occur on a moment-to-moment basis. No matter how skilled you are as a supervisor, you'd fail instantly and quite miserably. In addition to running your body without your help, this intelligence also powers your mind and the stories that make up who you think you are—and it doesn't stop there.

This same intelligence runs nature's cycles, pushing evolution along in ways that are not always predictable. Even though it is invisible, we feel its power in every sunset, the first blooms of spring, or the sight of a lioness protecting her cubs. This intelligence powers gravity, magnetism, and other physical laws as much as it does our circulation, digestion, and homeostasis, as well as our changing thoughts and moods. Nature never feels incomplete and merely submits to this intelligence.

We, on the other hand, feel incomplete because we don't realize that we are already whole and perfect. Knowledge of our true nature sets us free from suffering and fills us with bliss because we realize that not only are we whole, but also that nothing in creation is separate from us.

Even though the wisdom of oneness is ancient, modern quantum physics experiments are beginning to demonstrate that everything in creation is reflected in everything else.

In 1982 Alain Aspect, a physicist, questioned the previously held belief that nothing travels faster than light.[5] In a groundbreaking experiment, Aspect and his team discovered that subatomic particles like electrons seem to communicate with each other instantly across thousands of miles. These particles seem to have an uncanny knowledge of what the other is doing and mirror each other simultaneously. Aspect went on to describe quantum entanglement, where pairs or groups of particles interact in such a way that the state of each particle cannot be described independently; instead, the system must be described as a whole.

The Illusion of Separation

If you've heard of the famous double-slit experiment, you are probably familiar with the observer effect, which states that merely observing a phenomenon changes it. In this experiment, a series of electrons or photons (light particles) are fired at a plate with two narrow side-by-side slits. On the other side of the plate, a photographic plate is set up to record the behavior of the particles. It turns out that a particle will ordinarily act like a wave by passing through both slits simultaneously and produce a wave pattern on the photographic plate. However, if we observed the particle, it passes through only one slit to produce a different pattern.

Many questions come up when we think about this experiment. Does the unobserved particle split up or does it turn into a wave as it approaches the slits? How does it know that a pair of slits is coming? And how does it change its behavior when it is being observed? Are the observer and the observed one, with no separation in the first place?

The Hawthorne effect is a similar phenomenon, where the behavior of individuals being observed changes when they are aware that they are being watched. Consider, then, that all the thousands of patients in

---

5   A. Aspect and D. G. Roger, "Experimental test of Bell's inequalities using time-varying analyzers," *Physical Review Letters* 49, no. 25(20 Dec 1982): 1804.

clinical trials who know that they are being watched change their behavior; how objective are the results of these trials?

The problem with measuring phenomena (or results in clinical trials) is that we don't take into account that we, the observers, are also part of the phenomena that we are trying to observe.

Scientists now tell us that electrons and other particles remain in tune with each other across great distances, not by mystic communication but because their separateness is an illusion. Every cell of our bodies is perfectly synchronized to every other cell, each a blueprint of the whole. Everything in creation is, in fact, an extension of one greater principle. Thus, the tiny little subatomic particles in our neurons are intimately connected with every creature in the universe. Everything is a part of everything else.

Changing the Model

Almost on a daily basis, patients, friends, and family members ask me for my opinion about the latest fad diet, supplement, or exercise program that claims to be the next magic bullet that will solve all health problems. We as a society have found many things on which to blame our problems: carbohydrates, grains, fats, proteins, the government (or the "establishment," as one of my patients is fond of saying), the environment, the ozone layer, the tobacco companies, and so on. Rarely do we step up to take complete responsibility for the way we think, act, live, and care for our bodies.

When we begin to see that everything is a part of everything else, we stop believing in magic bullets. If you are chronically stressed about your job, angry about the government, and struggling in your relationships, heaping servings of coconut oil or yoga classes five times a week will be of little use. Your health and well-being will continue to suffer until you realize your part in your misery. When we see the intricate way in which all of nature is bound together, we stop blaming everything else for our challenges. We own our minds, actions, emotions, and thoughts.

When we own our minds, we set ourselves free. The lesser our dependence on external factors for our happiness and well-being, the greater will be the knowledge we gain about the interconnectedness of life. This is the great paradox. Our knowledge of the world around us is colored by how we see ourselves. As long as we take ourselves to be limited body-minds subject to the winds of change, the world will appear threatening or as something we need to exploit. When we see ourselves for who we really are, we see that the world is an extension of ourself and that it is filled with incredible joy and beauty. This unity or wholeness is the basis for the bliss model. Although modern science is gradually discovering the workings of the universe, bodies, brains, and minds, they were eloquently described thousands of years ago in a holistic model.

The Holistic Way

One popular mode of thinking with respect to preventing heart disease is to medicate everyone. Thought leaders puzzle over the fact that despite advances in treatment, we have made no dent in the prevalence of heart disease. Some have suggested "statinizing" drinking water (adding statins, the cholesterol-lowering medicines, to the water supply) or prescribing a "polypill" with small doses of all beneficial medicines to everyone. Fortunately, these ideas have not come to pass because we are now discovering that statins and other medicines are not entirely benign and have serious and disabling long-term effects.

Despite all the advances in technology, pharmaceuticals, and procedural/surgical skills, we have not made any significant strides in preventing heart disease. This is where modern medicine has failed terribly. This failure is the result of not understanding the connection between disease and the mind. If we are not motivated to change our lifestyle, we cannot prevent heart disease or the other chronic illnesses that make up the overwhelming costs in healthcare. Our lifestyle, in turn, is dependent on how we think and feel about ourselves, the world around us, and about health and disease. A holistic approach is direly needed to make strides in prevention.

Holistic care does not imply switching from synthetically produced pharmaceutical agents to herbal preparations or eschewing life-saving modern therapies. Holistic refers to *holism*, defined as "a theory that the universe and especially living nature is correctly seen in terms of interacting wholes that are more than the mere sum of elementary particles."[6] This approach to healing is to consider the whole person—the mind, the body, and everything that makes up that person.

This model excludes nothing—our jobs, our daily habits, what we eat, how we eliminate, how we think, how we process emotions, how we relate to others and the environment, what we take in through our senses, and how we see ourselves and the world around us. Disease is the result of a misapprehension in any of these aspects of our lives and arises from the default model, which separates the mind from the body and both from life.

Holism takes on a radically different meaning when we consider that the basis for all human suffering is also the foundation for health and disease. This consideration requires a change in our operating model, which we will examine over the next few chapters. However, in keeping with the true spirit of holism that doesn't exclude modern therapies, we will first explore the marvelous advances that have revolutionized the treatment of heart disease.

---

6   https://www.merriam-webster.com/dictionary/holism

Summary

- Your body has no ability to care about how hard you try to make changes and only responds to how your lifestyle affects the brain and hormonal pathways.

- Prevention and treatment in the default model assume that suffering is the result of disease.

- We are bound to suffer when we operate in the default model, where disease can threaten our identity and survival.

- Health in the bliss model is defined as a state of perfect balance in which all bodily functions are normal and the mind and senses are filled with bliss.

- The bliss model is based on the concept of wholeness, where everything in creation is part of everything else. Experiments in quantum physics seem to agree with this concept.

- Wellness is deeply facilitated through a shift from the default to the bliss model.

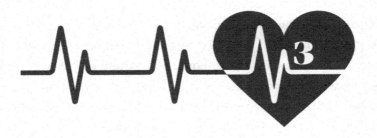

The
Magnificent Machine

Mark was sixty-five years old when he was wheeled into the emergency room on a cold winter morning. He had been shoveling snow in his driveway when a dull ache began in his chest, spreading to his back and left arm. Unable to catch his breath, he went in the house and called for his wife, Janice. By the time Janice came running from upstairs, he had collapsed on the kitchen floor. She called 911 and paramedics were at the door in minutes—they shocked Mark's heart to revive him, inserted a breathing tube, and rushed him to the hospital. The electrocardiogram (EKG) they performed in the ambulance showed that Mark was having a heart attack. His heart muscle cells were choking, being deprived of oxygen.

The heart is a pump. Like any other mechanical pump, it needs fuel to do its job. The heart's fuel is oxygen, which is supplied by the three coronary arteries that lie on its surface. If any one of these arteries suddenly becomes blocked, a part of the pump no longer gets oxygen and starts dying. Starved of oxygen, a part of Mark's heart began to die when he was snow shoveling, stimulating the nerves to call out in panic as pain.

The heart needs electricity to function, which is provided by a special-ized network of fibers within the heart muscle. When a part of the heart muscle begins to die off, the electrical fibers in that area short-circuit. By the time Mark came inside the house, the system had shorted and his heart had gone into an erratic rhythm and then came to a standstill.

Blood vessels coming to the heart are called veins and those leaving the heart are called arteries. The veins bring back deoxygenated blood to the heart, with carbon dioxide and wastes released by cells throughout the body. This blood is pumped into the lungs—we breathe out the car-bon dioxide, and the oxygen we breathe in is taken up by the blood. This oxygenated blood is brought back to the heart, which pumps it to the rest of the body, including the brain, through the aorta. Brain cells need oxygen even more urgently than heart cells—when Mark's heart stopped, his brain became oxygen-starved and he lost consciousness. Revived by the electrical shock that the paramedics provided, his heart restarted, but the blockage in the coronary artery continued to starve the heart muscle of oxygen.

When the ambulance arrived at the hospital, Mark was immediately rushed off to the heart catheterization laboratory, where doctors opened up the blockage. As he was wheeled into the intensive care unit, the car-diologist spoke with Janice about her husband's condition. Exhausted and scared, she wanted to know what had happened. Her husband had had no signs of having a heart problem. In fact, his family doctor had given him a clean bill of health only a month earlier. The cardiologist sat down with her to explain the underlying process of Mark's condition, which is known as atherosclerosis.

Atherosclerosis

Commonly called "hardening of the arteries," atherosclerosis is the pro-cess that results in blockages in arteries resulting in "attacks" such as acute coronary syndrome (heart attack), stroke (brain attack), or peripheral arterial disease (leg attack).

Atherosclerosis is a complex process that begins in childhood and continues undetected for decades. Several factors contribute to the formation of atherosclerotic blockages in the coronary arteries, which arise from the aorta and sit like a crown above the heart (*corona* in Greek translates to "crown"). Blood is ejected from the left ventricle into the aorta at a high velocity. When the heart relaxes, the blood in the aorta flows back into the coronary arteries. This high pressure creates turbulence in the flow of blood, creating tiny tears in the lining of the arteries. Exposure to toxins like cigarette smoke, high blood sugar, and unhealthy diet, as well as psychological stress, lead to an inflammatory response in the damaged lining of the arteries and cause abnormalities in the blood-clotting system (more on this in chapter 4). As a result, specialized blood cells known as macrophages in the blood rush in to deal with the problem.

You may remember from high school biology that there are three types of circulating blood cells: red blood cells (RBCs) that are responsible for transporting oxygen to the cells, white blood cells (WBCs) that fight infection and inflammation, and platelets that play a key role in blood clotting. Macrophages are a specific subgroup of WBCs that drive the formation of atherosclerotic plaques, or hardened areas in the artery walls. Macrophages are like vacuum cleaners, eating up and digesting dying or dead cells, germs, cancer cells, foreign substances, and anything the body needs to get rid of. They help maintain immunity and fight off illness. With this intent, they enter the walls of the arteries through the damaged lining and start to "eat up" the lipids (fats) that have leaked in. When such cells are viewed under the microscope, they appear like foam or bubbles and are called foam cells. These foam cells accumulate in the area of the plaque.

The plaque is separated from the blood flowing through the artery by a layer of cells that form a cap over it. When the cap is thin, it can be provoked by various triggers such as physical exertion, a big meal, cigarette smoke, sexual intercourse, drugs such as cocaine, emotional trauma, or even the natural rhythm of cortisol and other hormones. Janice reported that Mark did not exercise regularly; shoveling snow on a cold day when we are not used to physical exertion is enough to aggravate a plaque with a thin cap. Provoked by the sudden exertion, the cap over Mark's plaque broke off, exposing its irritating contents to the blood flowing in the artery. Immediately, the platelets in his blood rushed in to form a blood clot over the plaque to try to seal it off. They succeeded—at a cost. The clot blocked the artery entirely, preventing oxygen in the blood from getting to the heart muscle.

Complete filling up of the arterial lumen causes a heart attack that is often fatal. In fact, nearly one-third of individuals having this type of a heart attack never make it to the hospital. Mark had been fortunate that the paramedics arrived within minutes and were able to jumpstart his heart back to life. At this point in the explanation, Janice's concern grew. She began to worry—if Mark had such a serious condition, why did he not have symptoms? What should they have looked out for?

Symptoms of Heart Disease

There is a wide spectrum for symptoms and how people present with heart disease. The most common symptom of heart attacks is chest pain or discomfort, as Mark had. The discomfort can be anywhere above the belly button and feel like a pressure, an ache, or pins and needles, and it can travel from the chest to the jaw, arm, back, or neck. Sometimes the discomfort occurs only in these areas and not in the chest. A common symptom of heart disease is shortness of breath with or without chest discomfort. Women tend to have more atypical symptoms compared to men, with more shortness of breath, fatigue, heart racing, or a general sense of not feeling well.

The combination of a sudden onset of symptoms along with evidence of heart muscle damage on electrocardiogram (EKG) and blood tests is called acute coronary syndrome, a fancy way for saying heart attack. A heart attack produces sudden symptoms, but this is not the only way a plaque announces itself.

Quite often plaques gradually build up in the artery to produce a blockage. When this happens, symptoms come on only with exertion but not while resting. Exertion is any activity that makes the heart require more oxygen to do its work, including physical activity, physical exercise, or emotional stress, all of which make the heart work harder. The blocked artery can't provide enough oxygen to the heart when its workload increases, resulting in symptoms of chest discomfort, known as angina. When this happens over weeks or months, it is called chronic stable angina.

Janice confirmed that Mark had none of these symptoms leading up to the heart attack. This is not uncommon; the very first sign of a heart problem in nearly 40 percent of men and 60 percent of women is what we call sudden cardiac death. Mark was part of this statistic, where his heart stopping within minutes of feeling unwell was his first symptom. This brings up a valid concern. How can we detect heart disease before such a potentially fatal event happens? How had Mark gotten a "pass" on his stress test just a month before his heart attack?

Detection of Coronary Heart Disease

We have many tools at our disposal to detect coronary artery disease. The type of test we would have selected for Mark would depend entirely on whether he was having symptoms or not. If he had complained of chest discomfort, shortness of breath, or other symptoms while exercising, we would have recommended a stress test.

Stress Tests

A stress test is called that because it is meant to bring on symptoms and signs of a blockage. Since gradually built-up blockages bring on symptoms with exercise or exertion, stress tests mimic such conditions. When we exert ourselves, our heart rate and blood pressure go up, along with a constellation of changes in the body, to adapt to the workload.

There are many different types of stress tests, based on the type of stimulus we provide for changes to occur in the body. Most often, doctors prefer the type where you exercise on a treadmill since this gives us information on how your heart and vascular system function as you go about your daily life. If you cannot exercise because of joint or other problems, a stress test using medications that simulate exercise by increasing heart rate or blood flow is recommended. We can take pictures of the heart as part of the stress test, which can give us additional information regarding the location of the blockage.

All stress tests can only pick up severe blockages, usually those that are more than 70 percent. Like Mark, many of us may have less-than-severe blockages that don't show up on stress tests. The thin fibrous cap of the plaque breaks off during times of unusual (or usual) physical, mental, or emotional stress when the artery becomes suddenly blocked, which causes a heart attack. Stress tests help us infer the severity and location of a blockage. To look directly into the arteries we will need a different test.

Coronary Angiography

The radical revolution in heart disease treatment began in the late 1920s when Werner Forssmann, a surgical resident in a small German town, inserted a catheter into a vein in his arm all the way to the heart, injected dye into it, and took an X-ray to see where the catheter was. He won the Nobel Prize in medicine almost thirty years later, and his work set the stage for others to use catheterization for diagnosis and therapy of heart disease.

Modern cardiology is unthinkable without his contribution, even though the medical community at the time thought that what he did was absolutely insane.

Coronary arteries can be looked at directly with angiography. There are two ways to do this: heart catheterization, or a CT scan. Both techniques look at the coronary arteries directly. Heart catheterization is an invasive procedure where thin, strawlike tubes called catheters are inserted through an artery in the groin, wrist, or arm and into the aorta. Once the catheter reaches the opening of the coronary artery, a dye is injected and the shadow of the dye filling the artery gives us information on blockage presence and severity. Angiography with a CT scan uses the same dye as in heart catheterization. However, the dye is injected into an arm vein through an intravenous (IV) line, and pictures are taken as you lie on a table that passes through a doughnut-like machine.

We choose a catheterization or a CT scan depending on your history. If it sounds like there is a definite probability of your having a severe blockage, then we recommend a catheterization, but if we are not entirely convinced, we prefer a CT scan. A CT scan is a great test to reassure us when you don't have blockages. On the other hand, if there are severe blockages found on the CT scan, you would still need heart catheterization.

Detecting Blockages When You Don't Have Symptoms

As we have seen with Mark, a stress test didn't help, and he didn't qualify for angiography because he had no symptoms. This is one of the biggest problems in modern medicine, where the detection of a serious disease when symptoms have not yet begun is a great challenge. In heart disease, some selected tests that have been found to be useful are inflammatory markers in the blood (such as C-reactive protein, or CRP), ultrasound of the neck arteries, and a calcium-scoring CT of the heart.

Of all these tests, the detection of calcium by a heart CT has been shown to be the most useful to predict the risk of having a heart attack or dying from heart disease over the next ten years. However, we are still not clear if everyone in the community or only certain individuals with specific risk factors would benefit from having this test, since we don't know if this approach will definitely help us reduce heart attacks or deaths. Most importantly, it isn't clear if any of these tests can motivate us to change our habits to prevent this widespread disease.

How Bad Is the Situation, Really?

In the US alone, the burden of chronic diseases and conditions is staggering. Heart disease, stroke, diabetes, cancer, arthritis, and obesity are the most common, most expensive, and most preventable of all health problems.[7] Seven of the top ten causes of death in 2010 were chronic diseases. Two of these chronic diseases—heart disease and cancer—together accounted for nearly half of all deaths.

---

7   Centers for Disease Control and Prevention (CDC), "Chronic Disease Overview," https://www.cdc.gov/chronicdisease/overview/index.htm.

Every year the American Heart Association works with the Centers for Disease Control and Prevention and the National Institutes of Health to provide a statistical update on the current trends in heart and vascular disease (such as stroke), as well as the risk factors for these conditions. This extensive data is difficult to mine and organize and is a task that takes years; thus "current" data lags behind by about three to four years. According to this data, one American succumbs to heart (and vascular) disease every forty seconds, a third of whom are under the age of seventy-five years. However, there *is* some good news.

Although heart disease still results in one of three deaths in the US, deaths from heart and vascular disease have declined by a whopping 30 percent over ten years (2000–2010).[8] Overall, there has been a 41 percent decrease in death from heart and vascular disease over the last seventy-five years, attributed to the development of new therapies and procedures, education, and early diagnosis.

Modern Therapy for Heart Disease

If Mark had collapsed with a heart attack just a half century ago, we would have prescribed bed rest and morphine—that is, if he made it to the hospital. His survival would have been shortened, and he'd be disabled for the rest of his life. Thanks to the availability of cutting-edge therapies, his artery was opened in time by a procedure known as angioplasty, which we will explore below. Two decades ago (and even now in many hospitals), he would have received clot-busting medicines to open up his blocked artery.

Clot-Busting Medicines

In the 1980s the development of clot-busting medicines began to improve the survival rate of patients having heart attacks. Understanding that blood clots clog up arteries and cause heart muscle to die, researchers took to using these medicines at the first sign of a heart attack, showing

---

8   A. S. Go, D. Mozaffarian, V. L. Roger, et al., "Heart disease and stroke statistics—2014 update: a report from the American Heart Association," *Circulation* 129: e28–e292.

a significant decrease in death and disability. Soon, not giving these medicines on time was considered malpractice. However, the next phase of treatment was going to change our approach even further.

Angioplasty

In 1977 Dr. Andreas Gruentzig, working in Switzerland, inserted a tiny balloon into a blocked coronary artery, and when he inflated the balloon, the artery opened up to restore blood flow. As expected, angioplasty took the world by storm and quickly became the preferred treatment for blockages in coronary arteries. Hundreds of clinical trials found angioplasty to be effective in relieving symptoms in chronic stable angina and saving lives during heart attacks.

Soon angioplasty was supported by using "stents," tiny tubes with mesh-like walls that act as a scaffold for the artery. Further research trials using various types of stents (including the latest ones that are coated with medicines to keep the artery open for longer periods of time) have demonstrated unequivocally that angioplasty and stenting are far superior to clot-busting medicines to treat heart attacks. This is how Mark's heart attack was treated.

Open-Heart Surgery

In addition to the clot-busting medicines and angioplasty that were groundbreaking innovations in heart disease, coronary artery bypass surgery was a radical procedure to treat blocked coronary arteries. In this procedure the heart is stopped temporarily and the body is hooked up to a heart-lung machine while the surgeon works on the arteries.

Arteries and veins from other parts of the body are used to "bypass" the blocks by hooking one end to the aorta and the other to the coronary artery beyond the blockage. In all of medicine, this is one surgery that has been shown to decrease symptoms and prolong lives, particularly in those with diabetes and blockages in all three coronary arteries.

After the angioplasty procedure, Mark was observed in the intensive care unit during his recovery. By the second day he was breathing on his own and was unhooked from the ventilator. On the fourth day he was sitting up in bed after a liquid breakfast and began to feel uneasy. An EKG didn't show anything, but Mark continued to deteriorate and became severely short of breath. The team ordered a stat echocardiogram, an ultrasound of the heart, that showed severe leakage of the mitral valve.

To keep the blood flowing in the correct direction, the heart is equipped with four valves: mitral, tricuspid, pulmonic, and aortic. Their function is to separate the chambers—the tricuspid and mitral valves separate the atria, the upper chambers from the ventricles, the lower chambers. The pulmonic valve separates the right ventricle from the pulmonary artery, which carries deoxygenated blood to the lung to be purified. The aortic valve separates the left ventricle from the aorta, which carries oxygenated blood to the brain and the rest of the body. If the valves become too tight, blood cannot flow easily into the next chamber. If they become too loose, they leak blood back into the previous chamber.

Mark's heart attack had damaged the apparatus of the mitral valve, making it too leaky. Even though the artery was opened with angioplasty, the damage had already been done and was showing up now. Blood from the left ventricle was flowing back into the left atrium; the sudden change in pressure overworked the lungs, which filled up with fluid and made him short of breath. He needed emergency open-heart surgery.

In the operating room the surgeons saw that almost the entire muscle apparatus of the valve was dead and decided that replacing the valve was the best option. Mark was wheeled back into intensive care eight hours later.

Implantable Cardioverter-Defibrillators (ICDs)

As Mark and Janice discovered the hard way, blockages in the coronary arteries and heart attacks can disrupt the electrical pathways and cause lethal heart rhythm problems. Mark eventually recovered and went home two weeks later. Three months later an echocardiogram was repeated to see if his heart muscle had recovered fully and if he needed an implantable cardioverter-defibrillator.

This life-saving device monitors the heart rhythm continuously and provides a shock at the first sign of a dangerous rhythm. Weak heart muscles have such disruptions in their electrical pathways that these dangerous rhythms can come on suddenly and unpredictably. Implantable defibrillators are some of the most useful innovations in modern therapy for heart disease. Mark's heart muscle had suffered extensive damage but had recovered with the life-saving procedures and the powerful medicines he was prescribed. He did not need an ICD.

Medications

Along with procedures and surgeries, advances in pharmaceuticals have radically changed how we treat heart disease. Among the many remarkable medicines are statins that lower cholesterol; beta-blockers that lower blood pressure, decrease the heart's oxygen demand, and improve heart function; angiotensin-converting enzyme inhibitors that prevent the heart from restructuring itself in a dysfunctional fashion and protect the kidneys; aspirin and other medications (such as clopidogrel, prasugrel, ticagrelor, and others) that prevent platelets from sticking to each other and causing blood clots; and many classes of medicines that help with angina.

In 2007 a groundbreaking large trial among patients with chronic stable angina showed that angioplasty was not superior to medical therapy in preventing death or heart attacks over nearly fifteen years of follow-up.[9, 10] This data is not entirely new; we have known for a while that angioplasty is useful only in relieving symptoms but not prolonging life. In contrast, optimal medical therapy helps with preventing heart attacks and deaths because atherosclerosis is a systemic process. This means that the disease affects all arteries in the body and not just some locations in the coronary arteries. Thus, fixing local blockages is of little use without treating the underlying process of inflammation and addressing the causes for it; more on this coming up in the next chapter.

---

9 W. E. Boden, R. A. O'Rourke, K. K. Teo, et al., "Optimal medical therapy with or without PCI for stable coronary disease," *N Engl J Med* 356 (2007): 1503–16.

10 S. P. Sedlis, P. M. Hartigan, K. K. Teo, et al., "Effect of PCI on long-term survival in patients with stable ischemic heart disease," *N Engl J Med* 373 (2015): 1937–46.

Latest Innovations

The therapies listed above are broad examples of the strides made in modern medicine and technology for the treatment of coronary artery disease. We now have the capability of replacing heart valves without surgery through a percutaneous approach, just like in heart catheterization. Open-heart surgery has evolved to become minimally invasive, where the heart need no longer be stopped for bypass or other types of procedures. Newer medications are becoming available to treat various heart conditions. Many heart rhythm problems can be treated with sophisticated procedures to ablate (block off) areas that short-circuit. As the field of modern medicine evolves, we will see exciting changes in how we treat and manage those with various types of heart ailments.

Other Types of Heart Disease

Coronary artery disease is the most common type of heart disease. However, dysfunction in any of the many parts of this sophisticated electromechanical pump can lead to disease. We can be born with defects that span the spectrum of heart structure and function. For example, the chambers can be incorrectly connected, holes in the heart can cause abnormal connections between the chambers, the coronary arteries can be distorted, the valves can have structural problems, and the electrical system can be abnormally hooked up, leading to dangerous heart rhythms and sudden death. Some of these conditions can be passed on through genes.

Infections and cancers can affect the heart, causing weakness of the pump and heart failure or death. The lining of the heart can become inflamed, infected, or calcified, which interferes with the proper return of blood to the heart. The process of dysfunction of each of these sets of conditions is highly complex. Our understanding of these processes is not complete and is constantly evolving with emerging research and evidence.

Since coronary artery disease from atherosclerosis is the most common type of heart disease that we see, this is where we will focus our attention. Mark was treated successfully for his near-fatal heart attack and wanted to know how this had come about and what he could have done to prevent it, which is exactly what we'll cover in the next chapter.

Summary

- Atherosclerosis is a process that results in artery blockage and is the most common cause for heart attacks and strokes.

- The most common symptom of heart attacks is chest pain or discomfort.

- A common symptom of heart disease is shortness of breath with or without chest discomfort.

- Women tend to have more atypical symptoms compared to men, with more shortness of breath, fatigue, heart racing, or a general sense of not feeling well.

- The combination of a sudden onset of symptoms along with evidence of heart muscle damage on electrocardiogram (EKG) and blood tests diagnoses a heart attack.

- For chronic stable angina, stress tests can be very useful to locate the site of a blockage.

- Coronary arteries can be looked at directly with angiography, either invasively with a heart catheterization or noninvasively with a CT scan.

- Heart disease, stroke, diabetes, cancer, arthritis, and obesity are the most common, most expensive, and most preventable of all health problems.

- One American succumbs to heart and vascular disease every 40 seconds, a third of whom are under the age of seventy-five.

- Deaths from heart and vascular disease declined considerably over the last seventy-five years due to development of new therapies and procedures, education, and early diagnosis.

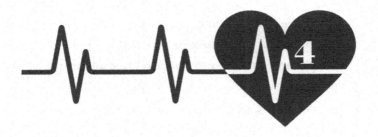

How Risk Factors
Turn into Disease

Decades of research and evidence have provided insight into the many risk factors for heart disease. When we decrease or modify risk factors, we can see a decrease in atherosclerosis, heart attacks, and death. Based on what we know thus far about disease and risk factors, they are divided into four categories:[11]

- Category I risk factors are those in which research has proven that intervention reduces risk. They include cigarette smoking, high LDL (bad) cholesterol, high-fat diet, high blood pressure, thick heart muscle, and high levels of a marker of inflammation in the blood known as C-reactive protein.

- Category II risk factors are those in which intervention is likely to reduce risk. They include diabetes, physical inactivity, obesity, low HDL (good) cholesterol, and high triglycerides.

11 J. M. Gaziano, *Global Burden of Cardiovascular Disease* in P. Libby, R. O. Bonow, D. L. Mann, D. P. Zipes, and E. Braunwald (editors), *Braunwald's Heart Disease: A Textbook of Cardiovascular Medicine* (Philadelphia, PA: Saunders, 2008), 1–22.

- Category III risk factors are those in which intervention may reduce risk, including psychosocial factors, high levels of homocysteine and lipoprotein(a), excessive alcohol (more than 2 ounces per day), and abnormal stress response of the lining of the arteries.

- Category IV risk factors are those that are associated with heart disease but cannot be altered: age, male gender, and family history with specific genetic issues, which is rare.

It is important to understand that these categories are based on what we have found easier to focus on. For example, it is easier to measure blood pressure and cholesterol than your psychosocial status. It is also easier to prescribe medications for risk factors than to counsel patients to change their habits that caused them in the first place, resulting in categorizing them in the above manner. It is exceedingly difficult to do large-scale trials of changing behavior and measuring such a change; in comparison, it is much easier to prescribe medicines to one group and a placebo to another and measure blood pressure or cholesterol. The above categories reflect the inherent limitations of evidence-based medicine that we overlook as doctors and patients.

Mark, whom we met in the previous chapter, had high blood pressure, diabetes, and high cholesterol, all of which were being treated with medicines. As he discovered, it is one thing to have risk factors for heart disease and another to have heart disease. The pathway from risk factors to disease involves a complex and intricate interplay of various chemicals and hormones whose function is to maintain homeostasis, or balance, in our blood vessels.

Endothelial Dysfunction and Inflammation

Endothelial Dysfunction

If you are an average-sized adult, you have anywhere between 1 to 1.5 gallons of blood circulating through your heart and blood vessels, which are lined by a single layer of cells called endothelium. Apart from your skin, your endothelium is the largest organ in your body, and it helps maintain balance in all your tissues and organs. Damage to this layer or imbalance in the chemicals it produces is known as endothelial dysfunction, which is the first manifestation of atherosclerosis.[12]

Your vessels are constantly adjusting to blood flow, plumping up or clamping down in various areas of the body based on what time of day it is, what you're thinking, how you're feeling, how high or low your blood pressure and heart rate are, and what the other organs (such as the kidney or liver) are doing. This delicate balance is maintained by the chemicals that the endothelium produces, the most important of which is nitric oxide. As long as your endothelial cells are producing a constant level of nitric oxide, your arteries remain healthy in response to your internal and external environment, plumping up or clamping down to maintain their tone. Moreover, as long as there is a normal level of nitric oxide in your arterial walls, your platelets don't stick together to cause clots and your white blood cells don't stick to the walls (see chapter 3). As soon as the endothelium becomes injured, however, an inflammatory process begins to heal the damage.

Inflammation

Inflammation is a normal protective response of the body to injury or harmful stimuli such as bacteria, viruses, environmental toxins, and irritants. Inflammation is your immune system's way of repairing and healing itself. Just as your skin heals with a scar when you cut it, inflammation in the endothelium initiates a scarring process when it is damaged by the various risk factors listed above. Quite simplistically, the delicate cells of your arterial walls undergo irreversible changes when exposed to toxins such as cigarette smoke, drugs like cocaine, excess cholesterol, sugar, homocysteine, lipoprotein(a), or triglycerides circulating in your blood or if you have blood flow disturbances because of high blood pressure, like Mark. With the onset of a proinflammatory process, certain genes

---

12 M. A. Gimbrone Jr. and G. Garcia-Cardena, "Endothelial cell dysfunction and the pathobiology of atherosclerosis," *Circ Res* 118 (2016): 620–36.

become activated and produce a variety of chemicals that are meant to stop the injury.

Most of the time, the injury is limited and the endothelium repairs itself. However, certain toxic stimuli such as certain types of cholesterol induce a complex process of permanent activation of certain genes. In this case, your endothelial cells become activated and start producing harmful substances known as chemokines. Chemokines in turn attract macrophages and other cells into the vessel wall. If there are high levels of toxins (such as cholesterol or sugar) circulating in your blood, the vessel wall becomes chronically inflamed, leading to atherosclerosis. We now know that coronary heart disease is indeed a chronic inflammatory process that induces the production of certain substances such as C-reactive protein that can be measured in the blood. Endothelial dysfunction can be measured in the vascular laboratory by a test known as flow-mediated dilation (FMD).

Is High Blood Cholesterol the Sole Culprit?

The role of high cholesterol in heart disease is a hot topic for discussion and controversy. In 2013 the American College of Cardiology and the American Heart Association issued updated guidelines on cholesterol management, where they recommend statin medications to lower cholesterol among many groups of individuals.[13] Some recent studies have shown that high cholesterol by itself does not cause coronary artery disease, calling for reevaluation of the guidelines. However, the little-known fact about statins is that they are potent anti-inflammatory agents, which might explain their beneficial effects in atherosclerosis, an inflammatory condition.[14]

---

13 N. J. Stone, J. G. Robinson, A. H. Lichtenstein, et al., "2013 ACC/AHA guideline on the treatment of blood cholesterol to reduce atherosclerotic cardiovascular risk in adults: a report of the American College of Cardiology/American Heart Association Task Force on Practice Guidelines," *J Am Coll Cardiol* 63 (2014): 2889–2934.

14 M. K. Jain and P. M. Ridker, "Anti-inflammatory effects of statins: clinical evidence and basic mechanisms," *Nat Rev Drug Discov* 4 (2005): 977-987.

The important thing to remember is this: atherosclerosis does not occur without endothelial dysfunction and inflammation. If you have high cholesterol but no endothelial dysfunction or inflammation, you are unlikely to get coronary artery disease from atherosclerosis. On the other hand, if there is presence of endothelial dysfunction and inflammation, even low levels of bad cholesterol are enough to cause atherosclerosis. Moreover, high cholesterol circulating in the blood can itself be toxic to the lining of the artery resulting in endothelial dysfunction.

While the risk factors listed above are the better known ones that lead to these deleterious processes, there are other lesser-known conditions that lead to atherosclerosis by inducing inflammation.

Hidden Risk Factors

Nearly everyone knows someone who had none of the risk factors presented here and still went on to have a heart attack. This is because there are a growing number of conditions that are being linked to atherosclerosis by their ability to cause endothelial dysfunction and inflammation:

- Inflammatory diseases, including autoimmune diseases like rheumatoid arthritis, psoriasis, and lupus, that cause vasculitis throughout the body, including the coronary arteries.

- Vitamin D deficiency, which has been linked to subclinical atherosclerosis and inflammation (although larger studies are needed to establish how it causes disease).

- Gum disease, which induces an inflammatory process in the whole body.

- Shift working, with loss of day-and-night cycles (as we will see in part 2).

- Air pollution, which is thought to be a major contributor to increasing heart disease in developing countries.

- Sleep apnea, a condition where you can stop breathing hundreds of times per night. The tongue normally collapses into the back of the throat while sleeping—if there is not enough room in the back of the throat for air to pass through (usually because of obesity), the brain does not get enough oxygen. Reflex mechanisms kick in to wake you up when the pressure in the lungs and heart go up from lack of oxygen. You can wake up hundreds of times every night without remembering it. The only sign you may have of not getting enough sleep is severe fatigue during the day.

- Hormone replacement therapy in women. While menopausal hormone replacement therapy has been linked to heart attacks and strokes, the link with oral contraceptives in younger women is unclear. Some studies have shown that women who use oral contraceptives have higher levels of inflammatory markers such as CRP in their blood.

In short, any condition that leads to inflammation is a risk factor for heart disease. As we move into an era of sophisticated research technology and personalized medicine, many more risk factors will be discovered, along with interventions and therapies that are effective.

Heart Disease in Women

Julie came to my office as a last resort. She had seen three other cardiologists for her ongoing symptoms of chest discomfort and palpitations. The discomfort was atypical, as it would come on not only when she was exerting herself but often when she prepared for bed at night. She had symptoms of "pounding" in her chest on occasion, usually associated with the chest discomfort. At fifty-three she was in the throes of menopause with hot flashes and mood swings. One cardiologist had told her it was all hormonal and that heart disease is a "man's disease." Two others had performed stress tests, which turned out to be quite normal for her age. They too had dismissed her symptoms, telling her it was all in her head. She confessed that she did not feel well and had an intuition that there was something wrong with her heart. I trusted her and sent her for a CT angiogram since her probability for significant disease was not high. To my surprise, Julie had a severe blockage in one of her arteries, and the other two had mild blockages. She underwent angioplasty and was started on appropriate medicines. All her symptoms went away.

For decades, research trials in heart disease included a disproportionately higher number of men. This led to practices in the field of cardiology that were based on lack of knowledge of disease in women and several misconceptions, including the view that it is a man's disease. Such practices led to almost exclusive focus on men with respect to preventive strategies and education. Statistical data demonstrates the downstream effects of those misconceptions: currently, more women die of heart disease than men (nearly half a million in the US alone).[15] Moreover, women have more complications after a heart attack, including the probability of having another one, death, and heart failure.[16]

The field of cardiology is in its infancy when it comes to understanding heart disease in women. We now know that heart disease causes more deaths in women than breast cancer. Although there was the erroneous perception that women are "safe" from heart disease until menopause, this has been refuted by data in the last decade. Risk for developing heart disease begins long before menopause. Moreover, treatments in post-menopausal women don't seem to work as well as in men. As with Julie, women have been shown to have longer time to diagnosis, less intensive resource use, and delays in seeking care. Women tend to have more atypical symptoms of heart disease, with more fatigue, sleep

15 A. S. Go, D. Mozaffarian, V. L. Roger, et al., "Heart disease and stroke statistics—2014 update: a report from the American Heart Association," *Circulation* 129 (2014): e28–e292.

16 C. N. Bairey Merz, L. J. Shaw, S. E. Reis, et al., "Insights from the NHLBI-Sponsored Women's Ischemia Syndrome Evaluation (WISE) Study, Part II: gender differences in presentation, diagnosis, and outcome with regard to gender-based pathophysiology of atherosclerosis and macrovascular and microvascular coronary disease," *J Am Coll Cardiol* 47 (2006): S21–9.

disturbance, shortness of breath, and pain or discomfort that is not in the chest area.[17]

To complicate things further, traditional tests that focus on identifying blockages are not as accurate in women. Newer tests like calcium scoring and CT angiography seem to be as efficacious in women as in men. However, these tests expose women to X-rays that can be associated with breast and other cancers over their lifetimes. The diagnosis of heart disease in women is also strongly affected by the presence of psychological symptoms. As was the case with Julie, investigators in one study demonstrated that physicians displayed a significant gender bias with respect to diagnosis of heart disease, particularly if a woman presented with added symptoms of stress. On the other hand, men's symptoms were assumed to be "real" heart disease whether or not they presented with stress or anxiety.[18]

Risk factors seem to affect women differently than men. For instance, diabetic women have higher rates of death compared to diabetic men.[19] Even though some of these differences can be explained by the fact that women present at an older age and have other risk factors, it is not the full story. Psychological factors seem to play a greater role in disease development and management in women. One explanation for the seemingly greater burden of symptoms in women despite having no significant coronary blockage is somatic awareness. Women have been shown to be more sensitive to internal changes, including physical symptoms, emotions, and mental processes.[20] This is one explanation for why depression and anxiety are more common in women.

17 J. C. McSweeney, M. Cody, P. O'Sullivan, K. Elberson, D. K. Moser, and B. J. Garvin, "Women's early warning symptoms of acute myocardial infarction," *Circulation* 108 (2003): 2619–23.

18 G. R. Chiaramonte and R. Friend, "Medical students' and residents' gender bias in the diagnosis, treatment, and interpretation of coronary heart disease symptoms," *Health Psychol* 25 (2006): 255–66.

19 A. M. Kanaya, D. Grady, and E. Barrett-Connor, "Explaining the sex difference in coronary heart disease mortality among patients with type 2 diabetes mellitus: a meta-analysis," *Arch Intern Med* 162 (2002): 1737–45.

20 C. D. Warner, "Somatic awareness and coronary artery disease in women with chest pain," *Heart Lung* 24 (1995): 436–43.

Habits That Kill

Nearly half of all adults have one or more chronic health conditions, and one in four have two or more chronic ailments.[21] When we look at risk factors for heart disease and other chronic illnesses, it is striking to note how many are preventable. Studies have shown that four lifestyle habits cause most illness and early death related to all chronic diseases—lack of exercise, poor nutrition, tobacco use, and drinking too much alcohol.

Nearly half of the adults in the US have at least one of the following major risk factors for heart disease or stroke: uncontrolled high blood pressure, uncontrolled high LDL (bad) cholesterol, or current smoking.[22] Nine out of ten adults consume too much sodium, increasing the risk for high blood pressure.[23] One in five adults smoke cigarettes; cigarette smoking accounts for nearly half a million deaths every year in the US alone. Drinking too much alcohol is responsible for nearly 100,000 deaths each year.

These statistics have serious implications on how a nation spends its resources. In the US, most healthcare costs are related to chronic illnesses and the health-risk behaviors that cause them. For instance, the Centers for Disease Control estimated that in 2010 alone, the total costs of heart disease and stroke (both of which are caused by poor health habits and are largely preventable) were nearly $315 billion![24] Not only do these conditions cost a nation its economic (and other) resources, but they also result in decreased productivity and absence from work. In 2012 the cost of decreased productivity was $69 billion due to diabetes and $47 billion due to arthritis. From 2009–2012 loss of productivity was estimated at $156 billion due to smoking and $224 billion due to excessive alcohol

21 B. W. Ward, J. S. Schiller, and R. A. Goodman, "Multiple chronic conditions among US adults: a 2012 update," *Prev Chronic Dis* 11 (2014): E62.

22 C. D. Fryar, T. C. Chen, and X. Li, "Prevalence of uncontrolled risk factors for cardiovascular disease: United States, 1999–2010," *NCHS Data Brief* 2012: 1–8.

23 M. E. Cogswell, Z. Zhang, A. L. Carriquiry, et al., "Sodium and potassium intakes among US adults: NHANES 2003–2008," *Am J Clin Nutr* 96 (2012): 647–57.

24 A. S. Go, D. Mozaffarian, V. L. Roger, et al., "Heart disease and stroke statistics—2014 update: a report from the American Heart Association," *Circulation* 129 (2014): e28–e292.

consumption. It is not surprising that our habits have everything to do with our state of health. It is surprising how they enslave us.

Take the example of Jack, who was forty-two when he had his first heart attack. When I met him, he had been treated for the heart attack a month earlier with angioplasty. He worked hard at a job that involved physical labor and long hours, indulging in heavy drinking and chain smoking to keep his stress under control. In the early hours of a chilly fall morning, he experienced chest pain while camping in the woods with his wife. He knew he was having a heart attack because of his familiarity with the disease. His older brother had suffered his first heart attack in his thirties, followed by multiple stents, bypass surgeries, blockages in his legs that required amputations, and, finally, a heart transplant. Jack's mother had a heart attack in her fifties, requiring several procedures over the next twenty years. Jack was no stranger to heart disease or its risk factors. When we talked, he knew he was drinking too much and that his smoking was a big problem. He knew his diet was poor and that his stress was getting the better of him. In fact, Jack knew more about the detrimental effects of his habits than many doctors, yet he was unable to change his habits. This is where the mind comes in.

While we do not know all the risk factors for heart disease (or for any other condition, for that matter), modern medicine has overlooked the most significant contributing factor of our health and well-being: the mind. In fact, emerging data in the default model is beginning to reveal what the bliss model has maintained all along: that how we process sensory information and how we think and feel have a direct effect on heart health. In the next chapter we will explore the elusive body-mind connection and the brain-hormone pathways that keep us locked in unhealthy habits, as Jack's example reveals.

Summary

- Well-known risk factors for heart disease include age, male gender, family history (associated with specific genes, which is rare), cigarette smoking, high LDL (bad) cholesterol, high-fat diet, high blood pressure, diabetes, postmenopausal state, physical inactivity, obesity, low HDL (good) cholesterol, high triglycerides, psychosocial factors, high levels of homocysteine or lipoprotein(a), and excessive alcohol intake.

- Risk factors cause endothelial dysfunction, which is injury to the lining of the blood vessels. The injury initiates an inflammatory process, which becomes chronic in atherosclerosis.

- The lesser-known risk factors of heart disease are inflammatory diseases, vitamin D deficiency, gum disease, shift working, air pollution, sleep apnea, and hormone replacement therapy in women.

- More women die of heart disease than men and tend to have more atypical symptoms, with more fatigue, sleep disturbance, shortness of breath, and pain or discomfort that is not in the chest area.

- Risk factors seem to affect women differently than men, and psychological factors seem to play a greater role in disease development and management in women.

- Studies have shown that four lifestyle habits cause most illnesses and early death related to all chronic diseases: lack of exercise, poor nutrition, tobacco use, and drinking too much alcohol.

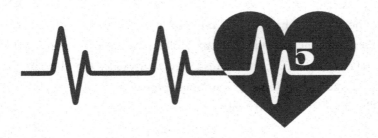

The Pathways of the
Body-Mind Connection

Centuries ago, doctors believed that emotions were linked to physical maladies, and it was not uncommon to prescribe a seaside vacation to recuperate from illness. Emotions lost their place as causative factors for diseases with the discovery of bacteria, viruses, and toxins. With exciting technological advances, the default model became stronger, with an exclusive focus on disease instead of the person with the disease. In the last few decades, the effects of emotional and psychological states on physical health have reemerged with stronger research and logic. The description of the pathways of the body-mind connection can be traced to the experiments performed more than a century ago by a Russian physiologist.

In 1901 Ivan Pavlov had conducted a series of experiments in dogs to study salivation in response to a conditioned stimulus. Every time the dogs were presented with food, a buzzer was sounded. Soon, the dogs would salivate merely at the sound of the buzzer. In 1975 Dr. Robert Ader, a psychologist at the University of Rochester, was trying to figure out how long it took an animal to become conditioned to a response. He fed mice sweetened water along with a drug that caused severe nausea and was surprised to find that once conditioned, sweetened water alone caused several mice to have severe nausea and even die. He concluded that the stimulus had led the mice to become immunosuppressed, or weakened in the immune system. Collaborating experiments with Dr. Nicholas Cohen, an immunologist, verified his suspicion: the conditioned stimulus did indeed result in immunosuppression.

These pivotal experiments that revealed the intimate connection between behavior, brain and immunology gave birth to a new branch of science known as psychoneuroimmunology (PNI). Current PNI researchers incorporate psychology, behavioral science, neuroscience, immunology, physiology, endocrinology, genetics, genomics, and other sciences in their hypotheses. In fact, we stand at a time in history where modern medicine is at the threshold of entering a new era of understanding the complexity of the body-mind connection. Ironically, the "new" era is not new. It had been systematically brushed under the rug under the default model, waiting patiently to be rediscovered.

Neurohormonal Pathways

While the intricate details of the body-mind connection are beyond the scope of this book, it is crucial that we understand how the evolution of our brains has led to the complex interplay between the electrical stimuli between neurons (nerve cells) and the effect of those stimuli on the release of specific hormones. This interplay occurs on a moment-to-moment basis, not only in response to our environment but also to our thoughts and emotions. The neurological-hormonal (henceforth called neurohormonal) response to external and internal stimuli affects all organs, including the heart. This response not only contributes to the development of heart disease and other chronic illnesses but also determines how we cope with disease. In fact, neurohormonal pathways are the source of suffering and bliss. Once we understand our biology, we can begin to take the steps needed to convert the pathways of suffering into those of bliss.

Your neurohormonal system consists of the nervous and the hormonal systems. Your nervous system consists of the central and the peripheral circuits. The central nervous system (CNS) consists of the brain and the spinal cord, while the peripheral nervous system (PNS) is made up of the somatic and autonomic nervous system. Each part of your nervous system has evolved in perfect harmony with all the other parts and over thousands of years to serve your best needs, and it all begins with its basic functional unit, the neuron.

Your Hardworking Neurons

Neurons are specialized cells with the ability to transmit information in the body and have two ends that make them look like elongated stars. Dendrites are spiky extensions on one end of a neuron that receive chemical and/or electrical information from other neurons. If the signal received is strong enough, it creates an electrical impulse that travels down the cell's tail, called the axon; the longer the tail, the faster the transmission of information. At the end of the tail is a hairy tuft, which is responsible for conveying the information to the next neuron. Signals travel at astonishing speeds from one neuron to another, resulting in voluntary and involuntary (or reflex) actions and reactions. A neuron carrying information from muscles and organs is called a sensory neuron, while one taking information for action is a motor neuron. Between the axon of one neuron and the dendrites of the next neuron is a gap known as a synapse, which enables signals to travel at great speeds by converting an electrical impulse to a chemical one.

When the electrical signal reaches the synapse, it stimulates the release of chemicals known as neurotransmitters. Neurotransmitters are hormones such as dopamine, endorphins, acetylcholine, and norepinephrine, and, as we will see later, they are released in response to external stimuli as well as to our own emotional responses. These chemicals float over to the next neuron, where they are taken up by the dendrites of that neuron and any excess is quickly mopped up by the tuft. The next neuron converts the chemical information to an electrical impulse and passes it on.

Unlike the other cells in the body, not all neurons divide and reproduce after birth. Once they die, they cannot be replaced. One exception to this rule is the hippocampus, which is the area of the brain that is associated with emotions, learning new things, and memories. Recent research has shown that new neurons are formed in response to learning and changing emotional patterns well into old age. This is great news for us since it indicates that we are never too old to change our nonserving habits that lead to endless cycles of suffering.

Neurons are some of the hardest-working cells of our bodies. Not only do they work tirelessly to transmit information about our safety, security, and survival throughout our lives, but—along with neurotransmitters—they determine the particular traits that make us who we take ourselves to be. To understand how this happens, we need to take a brief look at the overall structure of the brain.

Your Command Center: The Brain

Consisting of nearly 100 billion neurons, our brains were built from the "bottom up," since nature prefers to add on to what it has already produced rather than re-create its efforts. Thus, as we examine our brains evolutionarily, we can see what parts were added over the ages.[25]

Reptilian Brain

Right above where your spinal cord meets your brain is the most primitive part, known as the reptilian brain. Together with the hypothalamus that sits right above it, the reptilian brain is responsible for basic functions of your body, such as breathing, heartbeat, sleep, and excretion. Your reptilian brain also regulates your immune and hormonal functions (much will be said about this in coming chapters), acting as the switch between your emotions and your body. You can see your reptilian brain in action if you have anxiety-related diarrhea or constipation or if you develop hyperventilation with stress or have trouble sleeping because you're worrying too much about your upcoming work meeting.

Mammalian Brain

Located directly above the reptilian brain is your limbic system, known as the mammalian brain. Known as the seat of emotions, the limbic sys-

---

25 P. D. MacLean, "Evolutionary psychiatry and the triune brain," *Psychol Med* 15 (1985): 219–21.

tem has developed in response to experience. It is called mammalian because reptiles don't have this ability to the extent that mammals do. Take a lizard, for instance. Its life is dictated by a drive to remain safe from predators, maintain its body temperature (since it is cold-blooded), and reproduce. Its brain doesn't have a great capacity to learn from experience; it runs on instinct. It doesn't have the ability to change its behavior based on past experience to the same extent as mammals. Mammals (including us humans), on the other hand, can learn from previous stimuli that caused a specific response and change course accordingly, thanks to the limbic system. The mammalian brain is thought to have been added on to the reptilian brain to make social order possible. It enables the formation of herds and groups, social dominance, the need for contact with other members of the herd, competition for food and mates, and parental attachment—all the characteristics that we have in common with other mammals. The limbic system is what makes us learn to respond to stimuli in certain ways.

We can thank the limbic system for all our conditioned responses (including Pavlov's dogs that salivated at the mere sound of a bell and Ader's mice that became nauseated with sweetened water, as we saw above). Your limbic system locks you in to particular responses to stimuli based on your past experience. This is why we can turn to ice cream for comfort or dislike someone instantly. You may have no conscious memory of the first time you created a response, which is usually in early childhood. When you have an aversion or attraction to someone or something, certain neurohormonal pathways are being lit up that link them to the past unpleasant or pleasant experience. Particular hormones are released in response to stimuli that act as an alarm system, telling us if it is good or bad.[26] These pathways ensure our social and cultural conditioning—this is how we learn to behave in ways that enable our survival and reproduction, the two most critical functions as far as our brains are concerned. These pathways make us constantly scan our internal and external environments to seek out the ones that feel good and avoid the ones that feel bad.

---

26 L. G. Breuning, *Habits of a Happy Brain* (Adams Media, 2015).

Human Brain

The top layer of your brain is the neocortex or what is called the human brain, which is much more developed than that of other mammals. Your neocortex is what makes you human, allowing you to dream big, solve math problems, predict what might happen tomorrow, sort out your finances, use words to convey what you are thinking, plan for the future, and control your actions. The surface of the neocortex consists of deep grooves and folds and is divided into the left and right brains, connected by a thick bundle of nerve fibers known as the corpus callosum.

Each half of your brain controls the movements of the opposite side of your body. In general, your left brain is more adept at logic, language, and reasoning, while your right facilitates music, expressing emotions, intuition, and creativity. However, both halves of your brain work together and with the limbic system to process the information coming in from the world around you and how you respond to it.

Your neocortex takes in the information, but your limbic system is the one that determines if it is good or bad. Your neocortex cannot produce the hormones that make you feel pain and pleasure; only your limbic system can. Your limbic system, on the other hand, needs your neocortex to give meaning to your experience of pleasure and pain. Without the neocortex, you cannot find meaning in your daily experiences, a quality that we humans thrive on.

The neocortex was added on to the mammalian brain to recognize patterns between the past, present, and future. It is the part that not only enables learning from past experience but also imagining how that might affect the future. This is where you learn to anticipate feeling good with ice cream or bad with certain "types" of people. This extraordinary ability of finding meaning in experience by linking to the past and anticipating the future is responsible for driving the evolution of technology, medicine, space travel, and world events.

Lobes of the Brain

Let's take a tour of the vast neocortex that controls the various functions of being a higher mammal. Your very large frontal lobe enables your ability to think of abstract concepts, control your movement, and use words to express yourself. In fact, your prefrontal cortex (the front part of the frontal lobe) is responsible for what we call "executive functions." This is the part of the brain that determines your personality, makes you differentiate between what to do and what not to do, allows you to fashion your actions and thoughts based on your internal goals, suppress them when they are inappropriate according to your social and cultural conditioning, predict what to expect, and learn from your past. The frontal lobe controls short-term memory, while long-term memory is coordinated by the temporal lobe.

Along with the hippocampus (remember that is the part of your brain where neurons can regenerate based on learning), the temporal lobe creates long-term memories, including visual ones. This is the part of your brain you can thank for memories from your childhood, travels, and experiences that help you remember faces, places, and things as if they happened yesterday. The temporal lobe makes it possible for us to recognize objects, and, along with the parietal lobe, to process sounds into meaningful language.

Your parietal lobe takes in the information from your various senses to integrate it into a coherent whole. It determines your sense of space and how you move through it, what the different stimuli such as touch, pain, and temperature on your skin mean, and what words and language refer to. It is also the part of the brain that allows you to see things in your "mind's eye," while your occipital lobe is associated with processing sight.

All the lobes work together to take in information from our environment and respond to it. What we see, hear, smell, taste, and touch is processed in the temporal, parietal, and occipital lobes. Memories are created via the temporal lobe, and through the executive functions of the frontal lobe that refers to those memories, we respond and act according to our social and cultural contexts. Of course, this is an oversimplification of a very complex process that is still being unraveled, but you get the point— your neocortex is what makes you a complex being. Let's now take a look at how your brain communicates with the rest of your body. For this, we will have to turn to your peripheral nervous system (PNS).

Your Automatic Transmission:
The Peripheral Nervous System

Your peripheral nervous system has two parts, the somatic and the autonomic nervous system (ANS). Your somatic system is under your voluntary control and consists of the nerves that connect your sense organs (eyes, ears, nose, skin, mouth) and organs of action (hands, legs, organs of excretion, reproduction, and speech) with your brain. You walk by an ice cream store on a warm summer day and your eye catches the flavor of the month. It is cookie dough, your favorite. You must have some. You walk in and treat yourself to a cone. Here, your eyes took in information to the neocortex via sensory neurons. Your limbic system, which has learned from previous experience that cookie dough is good, gave meaning to the information in the neocortex ("Yum, gotta have some!") and the neocortex registered it, sending impulses down motor neurons to walk in, order, pay, and take a lick of the delicious treat. Ahead, we will see how you first decided that cookie dough was pleasurable.

Your autonomic nervous system lies outside your voluntary control and consists of your hypothalamus, brain stem, and spinal cord. Recall that your hypothalamus is also part of your reptilian brain. This is because it determines the hormonal responses that are necessary for optimal body function. The ANS has two arms: the sympathetic and the parasympathetic nervous systems. One difference between the central nervous system (CNS) and autonomic nervous system (ANS) is that the CNS neurons connect directly to the organs, while those of the ANS have an intermediary neuron. The neuron from the brain connects to the intermediary, which then connects to the organ.

Picture this: you are driving along the freeway at seventy miles an hour when your phone beeps, indicating an incoming text. Without slowing down, you take your eyes off the road to read it. When you look up, the traffic has come to an unexpected stop. In an instant your pupils dilate, blood flow is diverted from the stomach and digestive organs to your arms and legs, your salivary glands freeze, and your liver releases its store of glucose. Without conscious thinking, you slam your brakes and come to a stop, narrowly missing the car in front of you. Only then do you realize that your heart is pounding and you're breathing fast. Meet your sympathetic nervous system, the actions of which are mediated by the hormone called norepinephrine. Its job is to spring you into action in what is called the flight-or-fight response. It floods the body and redirects your energy and resources to do what you need to do now.

In the face of danger, the body doesn't care about digesting your lunch or keeping your mouth moist. It needs energy to act, which comes from the spurt of glucose. The hands and legs that need to run or stay and fight need more blood, which is redirected from other organs. You need better eyesight: the pupils dilate. Your heart works harder to provide more blood flow to the body, and your breathing gets faster to take in more oxygen.

When you are relaxing after a big Sunday brunch with nothing pressing to do, you can get a feel for your parasympathetic nervous system. Its main job is to digest your food and allow your body to rest. The neurotransmitter responsible for the rest-and-digest response is called acetylcholine, which stimulates the digestive organs to work, lowers heart rate and blood pressure, and constricts the pupils and the airways since you don't need to see particularly well or breathe as hard for this function.

Although the ANS functions well in times of stress to ensure your survival, there is a caveat. Chronic stress, as we will see in the next chapter, creates a perpetual loop of distress signals that have a direct impact on the heart.

Summary

- Psychoimmononeurology (PNI) is a branch of science that examines correlations between psychology, behavioral science, neuroscience, immunology, physiology, endocrinology, genetics, genomics, and other sciences.

- Our neurohormonal responses contribute to the development of heart disease and other chronic illnesses, determine how we cope with disease, and are the source of suffering and bliss.

- Recent research has shown that new neurons are formed in the hippocampus in response to learning and changing emotional patterns well into old age, which means we are never too old to change our nonserving habits.

- The "triune brain theory" looks at the brain as three parts: reptilian, mammalian, and human.

- Along with the hypothalamus, the reptilian brain is responsible for basic body functions, such as breathing, heartbeat, sleep, and excretion. It acts as the switch between emotions and the body.

- The limbic system, or the mammalian brain, is the seat of emotions and locks us in to particular responses to stimuli based on past experience.

- The top layer of the brain is the neocortex, or the human brain, which helps us find meaning in our daily life experiences and recognize patterns between the past, present, and future.

- The two important branches of the autonomic nervous system (ANS) are the sympathetic and parasympathetic systems.

- The sympathetic nervous system acts to spring us into action in the flight-or-fight response, which is mediated by norepinephrine.

- The parasympathetic nervous system acts in the rest-and-digest mode, which is mediated by acetylcholine.

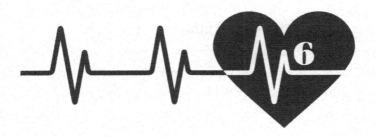

The Stress Cauldron

In my clinical practice, I routinely ask patients about their stress levels. It isn't uncommon for many patients to say they have no more than "the usual" amount of stress in their lives. When I ask them to explain further, they will go on to describe their sixteen-hour workdays, teenage kids going through difficult transitions, challenging relationships, sleepless nights, dependence on caffeine, chronic fatigue, heartburn, and other vague symptoms related to being "on the run." Most people think of stress as the acute kind that occurs with a catastrophic event like the loss of a loved one and assume that the ennui of daily life is normal for anyone living in modern society.

While it is true that there is "good stress" and "bad stress," the body doesn't differentiate between the stress of highly challenging life circumstances, such as extreme poverty or living in a warzone, from the kind described above. In this chapter I will explain why your body takes them to be the same and how the neurohormonal pathways that evolved to help us survive and thrive are also the harbingers of stress.

Your brain and hormonal system evolved primarily to ensure your survival and the propagation of your genes. Hormones ensuring our survival and reproduction evolved in parallel with our brains, in a "bottom-up" fashion.

Survival and Reproduction:
The Only Things That Matter

Imagine that you are among the first humans that learned to use fire and tools. On the vast savannah that is your home, you are preoccupied with staying alive and procuring food. You need to have the ability to immediately detect threats to your survival and act on it. Your reptilian brain was designed to do just that. It acts purely on instinct and has no ability to remember and learn from the past, which is the function of the mammalian brain, or the limbic system. The limbic system consists of several areas of the brain, including the hypothalamus and the amygdala, which work together in forming an emotional response to situations. This arrangement gave us a huge survival advantage since learning from the past and storing the information for future reference enables much quicker responses to animals that are bigger and have much more keenly developed senses than us.

How we react and what type of emotional charge is associated with particular situations is a complex phenomenon that occurs in early childhood and is facilitated by certain neurohormonal pathways. The amygdala seems to play an important role in assigning an emotional charge to the situation, assessing it to be fearful, benign, or one to be exploited. When it detects a threat to survival, the amygdala sends a panic signal to a part of the brain known as the locus coeruleus and to the hypothalamus. The locus coeruleus floods the body with norepinephrine and the hypothalamus activates the pituitary gland, which lies directly underneath it.

Our neurohormonal pathways have evolved to ensure our survival and propagation of our genetic material. In the following sections we will examine how these pathways continue to play out in our current sophisticated lifestyles far removed from the jungles and savannahs that they helped us survive.

Evolution of Neurohormonal Pathways

The peculiar ways in which we behave, think, and feel have to do with the pathways created for specific functions:

Take Action

The pituitary gland is called the master gland because it controls the other endocrine glands, including the adrenals that lie on top of the kidneys, the thyroid gland in the neck, and the ovaries and testicles. When the limbic system registers a stimulus as painful or undesirable, the hypothalamus activates the pituitary gland, which in turn signals the adrenals to release cortisol. What do you need to do if you are roaming around in the savannah and become aware of being hunted by a big cat? You need to take immediate action, of course! Along with norepinephrine, cortisol diverts your body's resources in the fight-or-flight response to deal with the problem. The sympathetic nervous system jumps into action, diverting blood flow to the muscles, dilating the pupils, and increasing blood pressure and heart rate.

Fast-forward a few thousand years: you are no longer being hunted by a lion on vast plains. You're no longer fighting for survival on a day-to-day basis, but here is the thing: your neurohormonal system cannot tell the difference between actual physical threats (like getting out of the way of a hungry lion) and imagined ones (like how you interpret your spouse's response to your comment). It reacts to both identically based on how you learned to respond to similar situations in childhood when you learned to register pain.

Deal with Pain

Unlike other mammals, human brains are not fully "online" at birth. Even though our brains have all the neurons at birth, the synapses, or connections between them, are formed by learning through our unique life experiences. These connections are immediately imprinted by the limbic system as pain or pleasure. Imagine that you are a two-year-old toddling around the kitchen as your mother is cooking dinner. She is cooing and talking with you as she turns on the oven. She lowers the oven door and instantly there is a loud boom as flames pour out onto her outstretched hand. She screams in pain as your father rushes in to extinguish the fire.

Fast-forward twenty years: every time you hear a boom, your heart starts racing and you start hyperventilating and feel like you are going to die. Your conscious neocortex doesn't remember the incident from your childhood, but your subconscious limbic system does. At the time the accident occurred, your amygdala registered a particular emotional response, propagating electrical impulses to produce cortisol and take action. Now, however, your neocortex tells you that there is nothing you can do about the distant boom that scares you but triggers the same pathway.

Every time you experience the stress of the stimulus and struggle to put an end to it, the neurohormonal pathway is reinforced. It becomes progressively easier for the electrical system to fire in the exact same way and produce the exact same hormones. It has become a conditioned response. Depending on how you handle stress, cortisol levels come down in as little as thirty minutes or a couple of days. If you have many pathways that lead to the same response, your cortisol levels remain chronically elevated since the limbic system wrongly detects that there is always something that threatens your survival.

Cortisol and similar hormones create the unpleasant feeling that we call pain, which jumpstarts us into doing whatever we can to make it stop. Our very large neocortex that helps us take appropriate action has a peculiar trait: because of its sheer size, it can make a very large number of connections with our past experience and concoct dangerous "what if" situations. The brain associates current situations with past ones because these connections fire and activate the limbic system, which activates the release of cortisol.

Because of our ingrained need to survive, we tend to remember bad experiences more vividly than good ones. Although this trait gave our ancestors a survival advantage, it no longer serves us in the current era, where our limbic system pushes us with an urgent do-or-die kind of feeling even when our rational neocortex knows that we are not in imminent danger of death. The amygdala, which coordinates fear, is unable to resist negativity and suffering. This is what appeals to us when we search out the worst kind of tragedies in the news, read and watch dark material in books, magazines, and movies, and hold discussions of doom with others.

Negativity is a survival trait, except that it turns the body-mind against itself when survival is no longer an issue.

The inherent need for survival becomes apparent in other traits that cause us suffering, such as seeking pleasure.

Seek Pleasure

We don't learn only pain and stress responses as we grow up. We also learn the ones that make us feel good and flood us with pleasure. For instance, you may not remember the very first time you tasted chocolate. The sugar and fat in it made your limbic system register it as pleasurable and caused a surge of dopamine, the feel-good hormone. Dopamine is produced by neurons in several areas of the brain as well as in the adrenal gland, and it makes us seek out what is pleasurable.

When dopamine floods the body, the limbic system registers it as a great feeling and nudges us to seek more of it. However, dopamine doesn't last long in the body and breaks down quickly, taking the pleasurable feeling with it. So we seek the pleasure again and again. Dopamine's other quirk is that it makes us quickly get used to the stimulus. This is why the first lick of your favorite ice cream is much more exciting than the subsequent ones.

Seeking pleasure gave us an evolutionary advantage—sugar and fats in the face of chronic scarcity were important for metabolism. Seeking such foods fueled by pleasure ensured our survival. Similarly, the pleasure of sex ensured progeny, and the pleasure of having more notoriety or possessions ensured our hierarchy and bettered our chances for living longer.

Fast-forward to now, and dopamine continues to push us into endless seeking. We seek more and more of whatever the limbic system registers as good, be it chocolate, drugs, relationships, sex, achievement, fame, or wealth. Now, however, it is no longer about survival but simply about feeling good. My life, for example, was marked by constantly chasing academic success. Did I need to be so ambitious? No, but success felt good until I saw that it never lasted. In this mode of constant seeking, we are never satisfied with what we have and tend to live in anticipation of the future, when "things will be better"—as in having more of whatever we seek.

Endorphins are the other "feel good" hormones in the body and represent another example of our brains doing their job to keep us safe and alive. Endorphins are produced by the pituitary gland in response to physical pain. It evolved to allow us to escape danger by numbing us to the sensation of pain. You may have heard of a situation where somebody was gravely injured and never felt the pain until much later; that is the merciful action of endorphins. However, they are also produced with extreme physical exertion, such as in a "runner's high." While a good laugh or cry can also induce endorphin production, our social pain, disappointments, and hurts don't induce endorphin production like bodily pain does.

As with dopamine, there is a price to pay for this high. Endorphins are produced only if you push yourself beyond your capacity and to a point of discomfort. Like dopamine, greater and greater levels of physical pain are needed to produce a high. Originally evolved as your brain's way of keeping you alive, dopamine and endorphins have turned us into pleasure-seeking beings. They keep us on the edge by inducing what is known as "good stress," where we are turned on by the seeking of challenges in our daily lives—exciting things like promotions and new relationships and life situations.

The seeking creates temporary bursts of cortisol and norepinephrine that help us function in the focused mode (see chapter 5) and complete challenges we set for ourselves. Modern society thrives on this type of "good stress" (or eustress), since it propels advances in human achievements. However, there is a fine line between good and bad stress, since the dopamine that rises and falls makes us seek more and more of whatever gives us pleasure or a sense of fulfillment. Since we can never be guaranteed of getting what we seek, the neocortex sends "what if" distress signals that chronically stimulate the stress pathways. Pleasure-seeking becomes stressful.

Our innate drive to survive not only leads us to seek pleasure and avoid pain, but it sets us up for comparison and judgment in relationships.

Compare and Judge

Picture yourself again in the savannah a few thousand years ago. Not only are you struggling to stay alive, but you are competing with your tribe for access to food and mates. You lose if you snooze, and therefore you feel the need to dominate. When you become the dominant one in your tribe, the others show you respect and reverence and your limbic system registers this as a favorable thing, activating the production of serotonin. Serotonin makes you feel safe and that you are assured of having your needs met.

Fast-forward to current times: even though our survival is no longer dependent upon dominating the tribe, these impulses remain in our need to be seen as worthy, respectable, or admirable. Even when we don't verbalize it, our minds are creating a hierarchy and gauging where we stand. Like TV shows and politicians, we are always aware of our approval ratings. When we gain approval from others, the limbic system notes it as good and the electrical pathway releases serotonin. How we view ourselves depends on comparing ourselves with others and judging others against the standard we set for them.

Our societies are far more evolved and refined now, thanks to logic and reasoning arising from the neocortex. We don't bully our way to domination, where we may not gain approval and respect from others—we can't induce enough serotonin to make us feel good. Instead, we unconsciously strive to be on top, leading to an onslaught of stress hormones. Since the hypothalamus is always looking to keep balance, the brain is constantly assessing how to gain others' approval without producing too much cortisol. What we call self-esteem or self-confidence is often the good feeling that comes from subtly (or overtly) comparing ourselves. When we are assured that we are more fortunate or endowed in comparison, the limbic system recognizes it as a good feeling.

Comparison, judgment, and one-upmanship are the building blocks of modern society. From college applications to job opportunities, we are encouraged to outsmart others and come out on top. We push our children to recognition and better opportunities to give them an edge over others. We feel gratified with likes and comments on our social media posts and feel let down if nobody notices. Our mind automatically sizes up someone as they walk into the room. If our brains register them to be at a lower level, we relax. If not, we feel a vague sense of unease. The conscious brain has no idea why we feel the way we do, and often we can't even articulate it. The limbic system, on the other hand, is just doing its job of ensuring our survival and that of our offspring. As far as it is concerned, our genes have the best chance of propagation if we and our offspring come out on top.

What began as a survival mechanism is now fraught with stress because our evolved society makes us carry a social, cultural, and moral conflict about comparison and judgment. Our logical neocortex tells us that we are not supposed to compare or judge, which the limbic system detects as internal conflict, so it activates more stress hormones. Not only are we constantly comparing and judging, but we are also stressed about it!

As we see, survival is a complex physical, mental, psychological, and biological process. In addition to the above traits, survival in mammals (including us) is deeply dependent on forming social structures through the important trait of attachment.

Become Attached

Okay, we are back on the savannah struggling for survival, where we quickly learn that it is to our great advantage to band together. Not only do we stand a better chance of surviving the dangers of the terrain, but we can thrive when we cooperate. Our chances of finding food and mates are much higher in a group. Most importantly, a group ensures that our offspring get off to a good start by learning from our experiences, and for this we need neurohormonal pathways that ensure attachment.

The hypothalamus not only initiates hormone secretion by other glands but is also a potent endocrine gland itself and produces oxytocin, which is needed for you to feel attachment and bond to your family and children, to want to take care of others, and to find pleasure in social structures. Oxytocin is the hormone that makes us long for companionship. It makes us trust others, flowing from the neuron connections that make us feel good in our interactions. The greater the oxytocin, the higher the attachment to mate, offspring, and group.

Attachment is one of the significant advances of the mammalian brain over the reptilian one. The larger a mammal's brain, the lower the number of pregnancies a mother can have over her lifetime. Thus, she must do everything in her power to ensure her babies' survival so that her genes can thrive. Oxytocin fosters attachment and ensures our survival, considering how helpless we are as newborns. Attachment facilitates our learning from others, particularly our parents and caregivers.

Not only do our rapidly developing brains absorb vast amounts of information, but they are also equipped with mirror neurons, which fire in response to someone else getting a reward or punishment. For instance, we are less likely to touch a hot stove if we watched someone else do it and squeal in pain. These special neurons make us learn from others' experiences.

Fast-forward to now, and we see that these responses that evolved to ensure our survival are also sources of stress. Social living is fraught with many challenges, including competition, struggle for dominance, and the need to form bonds with the other members of the group, even when we don't want to. You are forced to tolerate your mother-in-law when she visits just to keep peace with your husband, even when she pushes all your buttons. Your mirror neurons make you feel miserable around miserable people because your limbic system triggers an alarm signal.

Not only do mirror neurons enable empathy, but they also make us band together in a shared sense of threat. Remember how our brains are wired to respond more strongly to negative situations (real or imagined) than positive ones? Add the effect of mirror neurons to our inherent need for social structures and we have the perfect set-up for cortisol-powered and fear- or hatred-fueled groups acting against others based on imagined threats to their survival. This is what makes us bond together in gossip, heated political and religious discussions, and shared likes and dislikes. Paradoxically, this cortisol-powered sense of threat harbors attachment. Belonging in a group is much more desirable even with all the stress, compared to loss of attachment and the drop in oxytocin that makes us feel miserable. We'd rather stay in toxic groups and relationships because the alternative is unthinkable.

Social structures also come with the potential for heartache. If our trust was challenged in early childhood, the limbic system stores it away as pain and infuses us with suspicion in future relationships. If our sense of trust is betrayed (in reality or imagination), the neurohormonal pathways of pain are triggered and the limbic system immediately concludes that this is a situation you must run from, either literally or figuratively. Stress hormones pour into your system. The neocortex, which is capable of logic and reasoning, weighs the options and draws conclusions about who to trust and whether you should trust at all. The limbic and hormonal systems respond accordingly, producing oxytocin or stress hormones in relationships.

Despite their challenges, social structures ensure our survival by ensuring the propagation of our genes through reproduction.

Reproduce

Let's return to the savannah again (this is the last time, I promise!), but now to a much earlier time in evolution. Mammalian females lose precious resources, including energy, with every pregnancy and childbirth, and because of the toll it takes on them, attachment to their offspring is assured by the production of hormones like oxytocin, as we saw earlier. It is a huge disadvantage for the female to be fertile all the time, considering her limited resources and her need to take care of her young. Cyclical hormonal regulation provides her with the evolutionary advantage of ensuring quality of offspring over quantity.

On the other hand, the male has no binding attachment to his young since much of the attachment in humans stems from social and cultural structures rather than being purely biological; he is driven to inseminate as many females as possible to ensure the survival of at least some of his progeny. Quantity trumps quality for mammalian males. In such a disparity, males are required to woo the females with the unique traits that tell her that he is an acceptable mate with good genes, which translates to greater chances for her offspring to survive. Not only must a male appear attractive to a female in the group, but he also must compete with the other males for her attention. The females, on the other hand, are not particularly pressured to attract males. These evolutionary differences between the sexes gives rise to dimorphism, where sex hormones act differently on males and females to give them their unique characteristics.

Estrogen is the main hormone responsible for dimorphism and is produced in both sexes. Estrogen produces permanent changes in developing male brains by establishing nerve connections in the neocortex and the limbic system, which ensure behaviors like aggression in adult males. Estrogen is also required for activation of adult male behaviors and works by being converted to testosterone in different parts of the brain. In females, estrogen production starts much later, when it can no longer masculinize the brain or induce male behaviors. Even though estrogen is responsible for the sexual dimorphism we see in the brain and behavior of both sexes, testosterone controls the intensity of masculine behavior in adult males during times when they are trying to attract a mate or fight off a rival.

Unlike other hormones that work on the outer membrane of the cell via gateways known as receptors, sex hormones can enter the cell's nucleus and influence the genetic material. The relationship between sexual dimorphism and behavior is highly complex because it is difficult to sort out whether we do what we do based on our neurohormonal systems or our social and cultural conditioning. In any case, the limbic system registers what makes a mate potentially more attractive, signaling the release of sex hormones that drive reproduction.

Fast-forward to now, and we are in the age where we can control our reproduction and choose our mates without immediate or imminent threat to our own survival or that of our children. However, social and cultural conditioning render sex as an object that fulfills the dopamine-powered reward pathways. As we have seen, seeking is stressful. Additionally, the complicated neurohormonal pathways related to living in a social structure and maintaining relationships affects how we view sex, which is not used solely for reproduction but also as a means of control, showing affection, and bonding. Our complex behaviors have a propensity to create chronic stress through the limbic system, which interprets various situations and activates the cortisol pathways.

Cortisol inhibits the production of the hormone in the pituitary that activates sex hormone production in the ovaries and testes, leading to low levels of estrogen in women and testosterone in men. Low levels of estrogen in the brain lead to greater susceptibility to stress and trauma in women, whereas higher levels of estrogen make her more resilient to stress. Insulin resistance and metabolic syndrome resulting from stress create further havoc in the ovaries, resulting in erratic sex hormone production with menstrual disorders and infertility. Similarly, high cortisol is associated with low testosterone in men, leading to fatigue, insomnia, and sexual dysfunction.

So there we have it: a very simplistic view of the neurohormonal pathways that mammals have developed to survive. Even though we humans have developed language and complex thinking thanks to the neocortex, our reactions and responses to life still arise from the relatively primitive limbic system. The neurohormonal pathways determined by the limbic system become established into how we think, feel, and act on a daily basis.

As we will see below, these pathways become superhighways, predisposing us to developing habit-based diseases and making it difficult to heal from our own nonserving ways.

Neurohormonal Superhighways: Creating Habits

Do you ever wonder why you do things specifically the way you do? Whether I'm reading a patient's echocardiogram or loading the dishwasher, I have "a way" to do it, which is different from someone else's "way." How does this happen?

Recall that unlike other mammals, we are born helpless and clueless. Our brains have all the neurons, but the synapses are formed through experience. When signals flow through the same neurons in response to pain and pleasure, those neurons develop a casing of protein known as myelin. If you're going to do the same thing repeatedly, you might as well discover a shortcut; this is exactly what the neurons do. Signals travel much faster with myelin, which develops through the same response repeated via the limbic system.

To become more efficient, new synapses are formed between the neurons that we use the most. Electrical signals jump from one neuron to another through chemicals. The first produces a chemical that floats over to the other that has its receptors, which are protein bits in precise shapes that fit the chemical molecule perfectly. If the same pathway is used again and again, more receptors are produced. If not, they decrease. Pathways fortified through acting and feeling the same way become superhighways. While the frequently used neurons become superhighways, the ones that are not used wither and die.

This does not mean we become helpless slaves of the limbic system. The situation is to the contrary, thanks to our very well-developed neocortex. Recall that the prefrontal cortex is the part of the brain that chooses. This part of your brain is continually weighing your options in response to the limbic system's automatic firing. This is where your decision to act on the impulse or to find another way rests. Once you decide, the limbic system responds to tell you if it is going to make you feel pain or pleasure. At the same time, different parts of your brain are processing information coming in from the world around you and within you. And it all happens in milliseconds, without your conscious effort or awareness.

If you give in to the impulse again and again, you help create the superhighway of habit. Driven by dopamine and the intricate web of hormones produced in response to the electrical pathways in the nerves, you seek the object again and again even when your neocortex advises you against it. The conflict between your reasoning and the habit superhighway creates stress—you know what is good for you, but you simply can't help it.

The Toll of Stress

By now, I hope that the connection between the brain, hormones, emotions, and behavior is becoming clear. How you think, feel, and respond to your situation results in the release of various hormones, triggering the autonomic nervous system (ANS) to fire in specific ways to affect the organs. Growing research in the past two decades is demonstrating the intricate ways in which the mind influences the ANS in the causation and progression of heart disease.

The heart is a pump, but it is much more than a pump. Along with the brain, hormonal system, ANS, metabolic and immune systems, the cardiovascular system helps the body cope with stress. If our outlook toward life is one of resilience, the spurts of cortisol and other stress hormones tend to come down in hours or days. However, when we don't deal with stress in wholesome ways, these hormones remain in the bloodstream chronically.

The brain cannot differentiate between acute and chronic stress and responds to the levels of stress hormones circulating in the blood by redirecting the body's resources for immediate action. Cortisol mobilizes glucose from the liver. The pancreas reacts to increased blood glucose by releasing more insulin. Over time, the organs are overwhelmed by cortisol, increased insulin, and the constant battle between themselves. The result of chronically elevated insulin is metabolic syndrome, with an increase in serum triglycerides and a chemical known as plasminogen activator-1 that increases blood clotting, and a decrease in high-density (good) lipoprotein. In addition, cortisol inhibits the immune response, sensing that fighting off infections can wait. Instead, it prepares the body to fight by increasing intravascular volume and rearranging fatty tissue.

Activation of the sympathetic nervous system by stress releases epinephrine, a hormone that increases the heart rate and decreases heart rate variability, an indicator of ANS health. If your ANS is healthy, your heart rate should fluctuate greatly from moment to moment. It should increase with inhalation and decrease with exhalation. It should increase when you exercise and return to normal within a few minutes of stopping the activity. This tells us that the two arms of your ANS are working as they should. Decreased heart rate variability is an indicator that the ANS is out of balance.

Both the cortisol and the epinephrine pathways cause endothelial dysfunction, and the overcharged sympathetic arm of the ANS stimulates the production of chemicals known as cytokines that activate the inflammatory response, as we have seen in chapter 4. With the presence of endothelial dysfunction, inflammation rapidly leads to atherosclerosis, heart failure, arrhythmias, and other potentially fatal conditions. In addition, stress hormones affect learning and memory through their effects on various areas of the brain, including the hippocampus.

The most dramatic effect of stress on the heart is seen in stress cardiomyopathy, a condition more commonly seen in women. In this condition, acute emotional or psychological stress causes patients to present with symptoms that are indistinguishable from a heart attack. However, no blockage can be found on angiography, and patients are found to have elevated sympathetic activation and stress hormones in the blood. The heart muscle is transiently weak, often regaining function over time. In fact, the discovery and exploration of stress cardiomyopathy has given more credence to the role of emotional and mental stress in heart disease.

Default Versus Bliss Model Perspectives on Neurohormonal Pathways

Notice that everything we have been discussing with regard to the neurohormonal pathways refers to the default model. Our quest for survival that drives our behaviors arises from taking ourselves to be the body-mind, which thrives on seeking pleasure and avoiding pain, struggling to find fulfillment in objects and relationships, and being distressed when these goals are not achieved. The body pays a price for this fundamental misunderstanding, turning against itself by using the very neurohormonal pathways that keeps us bound to the identity as the body-mind.

The bliss model describes these pathways from a different perspective, as we will soon see. In this model the various pathways of the brain are seen to result in mental modifications that obscure our true nature. They are like a covering of dust upon a mirror, which obscures our reflection. We become so enchanted with the dust that we forget what lies underneath it. We can rearrange the dust by turning bad feelings into good ones, but that doesn't change the fact that it is still dust and that it still obscures the mirror. Neurohormonal pathways are vital to our identification as the body-mind and keep us steeped in dualities such as good and bad, pain and pleasure, desirable and undesirable, and so on. Wherever there is good, we can be sure that there will be its opposite, bad. Hence, we can never successfully convert all bad to all good. Even if we succeed, as long as we are identified as the body-mind, we will eventually come face-to-face with something that causes us pain or distress. The solution is not merely to reduce stress or suffering but to examine the very basis of it, which is false identification.

Can this be done? Can we get off the neurohormonal superhighways or are we doomed to their effects? Let's see in the next chapter.

Summary

- Our neurohormonal pathways have evolved primarily to ensure our survival and the propagation of our genes and are regulated by the limbic system.

- When the limbic system registers as painful or undesirable, it activates the production of stress hormones such as cortisol to spur the body to take action against the perceived threat.

- The neurohormonal system cannot tell the difference between actual and imagined threats to our survival.

- Because of our ingrained need to survive, we tend to remember bad experiences more vividly than the good ones.

- Dopamine and endorphins make us seek pleasure.

- Comparison and judgment that make us rise to the top make us feel good by the release of serotonin.

- Oxytocin is the hormone that makes us feel attachment and form bonds with others.

- Estrogen is responsible for sexual dimorphism, or differences between male and female brains, traits, and behavior.

- When we act and feel again and again in the same ways, our pathways become superhighways, or deeply ingrained habits.

- Stress induces endothelial dysfunction and inflammation, leading to several deleterious effects on the heart and other organs.

- Neurohormonal pathways are vital to our identification as the body-mind and keep us steeped in the default model of dualities such as good and bad, pain and pleasure, desirable and undesirable, and so on.

- The lasting solution to our stress or suffering is not to merely change habits but to examine the very basis of it, which is taking ourselves to be the body-mind.

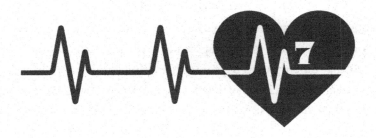

Can We Get Off
the Superhighway?

Most of our neurohormonal superhighways are formed before age seven and fortified during adolescence, when the brain works overtime to make sense of the world around us while being bathed in the sudden onslaught of sex hormones. If our existing highways make sense, they are cemented. If not, we struggle to form new ones, which is harder than in childhood. This is why puberty is so challenging!

If you think deeply about your emotional responses to situations, you'll find that they are quite similar to how you reacted in your childhood or adolescence. Your language may be more sophisticated and your reasoning may be more complex, but the fundamental emotional response is the same. Language and reasoning arise in the prefrontal cortex, which has made its connections over time, but your limbic system, where emotions are registered, was hard-wired much earlier in life. This is why kids who were bullies in high school grow up to be dominating and aggressive adults. Whether it is aggression or meek submission, the trait was cultivated because the limbic system registered it as being essential for survival.

Neuroplasticity

Even though our superhighways have been laid out from our repetitive behavior over years, it is indeed possible to change their courses. This is the trait that differentiates us from other animals. We have the ability to apply ourselves in such a way that we create new synapses and superhighways that take us from stress to joy. This remarkable ability of the brain to change course is known as neuroplasticity.

It is neuroplasticity that makes us learn new information throughout our lives and consciously make choices that are better for us. While superhighways are formed quite rapidly in childhood, it is a slower process in adulthood. This is why it takes us longer to learn a new skill or language compared to when we were younger. Remember that superhighways are formed through repetition. Compared to children, it takes us many more repetitions to change the course of our superhighways, but the good news is that neuroplasticity continues well into old age. We can keep changing our responses to suit our ever-changing circumstances.

Just as we are not stuck with the superhighways that we innocently built in childhood, we are also not bound by the genes we inherited from our parents. The recently emerging science of epigenetics is beginning to show us the shocking implications of this revelation.

Freedom from Determinism

Jenny was fifty-six years old when she came to my office for a second opinion. She had had her first heart attack at age fifty and told me with a bit of pride that she had seven stents. She became increasingly agitated as I interviewed her about her lifestyle and habits, stating that she was a "solid Midwestern 'meat and potatoes' type of girl", and that she had no time to exercise. She lived a sedentary but stressful life and was on a dozen pills for heart disease, high blood pressure, diabetes, high cholesterol, and anxiety. She asked me if I could prescribe another medicine for the occasional muscular pain she had in her chest. Reassuring her that she didn't need another medication, I reiterated the importance of lifestyle changes to prevent another heart attack.

She looked at me in disbelief and asked me if there was not enough evidence that her disease was genetic considering that both her parents and her three siblings had heart disease at an early age. When I asked her to review her family's lifestyle, she responded that all of them were severely overweight, smoked, never exercised, and were also "meat and potatoes" sorts of folks. She seemed unhappy to discover that we don't inherit just our parents' genes, but also their impressions—the way they live, act, think, and feel. As we explored in chapter 6, mirror neurons help us learn from others, particularly our primary caregivers. Our upbringing is reinforced by our caregivers' lifestyles and mindsets that we innocently adopt as our own. We don't have to rely on neuroscience to see if this is true. Instead, we can take a peek into the structure of genes to see if they really determine our fate.

Do Our Genes Determine Our Fate?

In the early part of the twentieth century, scientists discovered that hereditary information passed from one generation to the next was contained in chromosomes. These are threadlike structures in the nucleus of the cell that become most obvious just before a cell divides. When chromosomes were further dissected, they were found to contain two types of molecules—deoxyribonucleic acid (DNA) and protein. A quarter century later, DNA emerged as the sole carrier of genetic information. In 1953, based on the extensive work of scientists who had discovered its components, Watson and Crick proposed the double-helix model of DNA molecules that are made up of four nitrogen-containing "bases" (adenine, thymine, guanine, and cytosine, abbreviated as A, T, G, and C). A always pairs with T, and G with C. The sequence of the bases determines the amino acids (building blocks) of a particular protein.

The two strands of DNA are held together by hydrogen and are mirror images of each other. Thus, when the two strands separate, each contains the information to produce an exact replica of itself. The intermediary between DNA and life-sustaining protein is ribonucleic acid (RNA), which is a temporary copy of DNA that encodes various proteins based on the patterns of the bases.

When the world discovered how DNA works, it attained the superior status as the unchangeable principle that controlled our fates since the quality of an organism is defined by the natures of its proteins, and the proteins are birthed by DNA. This implied that the path from DNA to protein was a one-way event. Until recently, it was believed that our life experiences were determined by our genes but not the other way around.

Epigenetics

In the last decade, the science of epigenetics has begun to challenge the model that genes control our destiny in a one-sided fashion. Epigenetics is the study of environmental factors that turn genes on or off without altering the underlying DNA sequence. Studies show us that life influences such as stress, emotions, and nutrition can modify gene behavior. Not only do these changes affect the way our own genes work, but such traits can be passed on to future generations. Thus, the trauma your parents experienced not only could have altered their health, but if the modifications in their genes were passed on to you, you may experience the same kinds of health issues and also react to certain stimuli the way they did, even though you have no personal history with those stimuli. This is why we have aversions and attractions to things that we never experienced in our lives. Exactly how does the environment influence the behavior of DNA?

Remember that chromosomes contain two components: DNA and protein. The proteins were ignored for decades in the excitement of the discovery of DNA. It turns out that these proteins act as switches for DNA behavior by forming a sort of sleeve over it. If the proteins bind tightly around the DNA (via a process known as methylation), its genetic information cannot be expressed. Thus, you may have inherited a gene for breast cancer, but as long as the protein encases the gene, it is not expressed. An environmental signal is needed for the protein to change its shape and bare the DNA underneath, where it can be expressed. Thus, while DNA contains information, proteins control what information is actually expressed or switched on. The switch, in turn, is influenced by our lifestyles, habits, and how we think, feel, and act. Thanks to epigenetics, we now know that less than 5 percent of heart disease and cancer are attributed directly to heredity.

In one classic study in recent years, Dr. Dean Ornish and his team demonstrated that the activity of more than 500 genes can be changed through diet and lifestyle changes among men with prostate cancer. More recently they demonstrated that diet changes, a moderate exercise program, and stress reduction resulted in an increase in telomere length.[27] Telomeres are protective caps at the end of chromosomes. Recall that for a cell to divide, the DNA must first unwind so that each strand can duplicate itself. The duplication process is performed by an enzyme known as DNA polymerase, which travels down the strand to assemble the mirror-image strand. When it reaches the end of the strand, it stops because it cannot duplicate the part of the strand it sits on. Thus, every time a DNA strand is replicated, it is slightly shorter than the "parent" strand, and eventually the polymerase will begin cutting off essential information at the ends of the strands.

Telomeres provide a length of noncoding DNA whose loss will not affect the information contained in the gene. The length of the telomerase determines how fast we age as well as our susceptibility to illnesses such as cancer, stroke, heart disease, diabetes, osteoporosis, obesity, and dementia. Until recently we were under the impression that telomere length could not be changed. Epigenetic studies like the one above show us that this is not true and that our lifestyle influences the behavior of our genes. We can finally let go of the kind of paralyzing thinking that we saw in Jenny and be empowered by the fact that we can indeed rebuild our neuronal superhighways, which have a direct effect on our genes.

---

27 D. Ornish, J. Lin, J. M. Chan, et al., "Effect of comprehensive lifestyle changes on telomerase activity and telomere length in men with biopsy-proven low-risk prostate cancer: 5-year follow-up of a descriptive pilot study," *Lancet Oncol* 14 (2013): 1112–20.

Rebuild Your Superhighways
to Change Your Life

By now we know that our circumstances are far from being static. No matter how hard we try to control our lives, we never seem to succeed all the time. Sometimes we have what we want and at other times what we don't want. We constantly try to manipulate our life situations to find happiness. Driven by our dopamine-powered neural pathways, we seek the ideal education, partner, and job, never at peace with what we already have. Our neurohormonal system just doesn't let up and keeps us on the path of seeking throughout our lives. Once we have breathed a sigh of relief that our children are reasonably well-educated and have gone off to college, we feel the familiar nagging of seeking where we now want for them everything that we wanted for ourselves (and more). Worries about their relationships and jobs keep us up at night. Just as soon as our retirement party ends, we are faced with concerns about our grandchildren and whether they are being raised right. Then, as the wrinkles and grays proliferate, we are nagged by the greatest anxiety of all: our impending death.

Through all this, rarely do we stop to wonder if this dissatisfaction is our destiny. We look around, see that everyone is more or less in the same boat, and conclude that this constant dissatisfaction with what is must be normal. We live our lives constantly at war with whatever is going on around us since it never meets our definition of "ideal." It is not only the world that does not conform to our unique definitions of good and bad; even our bodies begin to let us down. We fall sick and develop disease despite the limbic system's protest that this is a bad thing. If we are not fighting the world, we are fighting our bodies and minds. Through it all, the neurohormonal pathways continue to do their thing, revving up the stress pathways that cause internal havoc.

At any given time we are ruminating about the past or the future. Pause for a moment and answer these questions. How many times did you have to re-read sections of this book because you were "somewhere else" when you first read them? How many times have you driven from point A to B only to realize you don't remember getting there? When in a conversation, how many times do you find that you've missed parts of what the other person is saying because you were not paying attention?

Now consider this: What were your thoughts about when you were not present in an activity? What is the constant mind chatter about?

Default Mode Network: The I-Maker

It turns out that only 5 percent of the brain's total energy consumption is for focused tasks such as reading or working on a project. Most of the brain's energy is consumed in the ongoing personal narrative that weaves together the various experiences of our lives into one coherent story. In other words, the brain uses most of its energy ensuring that you remain the protagonist in the story of your life. For this, you can thank your default mode network (DMN).

The DMN is a network of various brain centers that light up simultaneously when focused attention is not required. Consisting of three arms, it is the network that brain activity defaults to. The first arm is responsible for the personal autobiographical storytelling, or the I-making that is self-referencing (thoughts that revolve around why you like or don't like something and how these choices define you) and validates your own emotional state. Any time you are retelling your story in your mind, this network is active. The second arm of the DMN is associated with assuming what someone else knows or doesn't know, understanding someone else's emotional state, moral justification, assessing right and wrong, and evaluating the social standing of your family, group, or tribe. The third arm of the DMN is associated with recalling the past, imagining the future, and the ability to connect the two into a story.

The DMN keeps the I alive and well. The curious thing about the I is that it consists of fragments of information such as your likes and dislikes, your ancestry, and how you feel about your nose, body, job, spouse, children, or race. The I isn't one thing but a whole box of ideas about who you think you are. You collected these ideas over the course of your life and then built your identity upon them, and you've collected them because each came with a distinct emotional high or low that created particular neurohormonal superhighways.

We collect most of the ideas about who we are before the age of seven. The younger we were when an emotional signature arose, the more surely was a superhighway created. This is when we started believing things like "I'm cute," "My nose is too big," "I'll never be good at sports," or "I'm a good musician." In adolescence our superhighways were reinforced as we added on to our existing beliefs, strengthened them, and added new ideas based on more complex concepts like religion and politics. Unlike in childhood, stories around our ideas become more complex in adolescence. As young adults we embellish our beliefs with more elaborate and sophisticated stories. The I is created through the self-referencing part of the DMN, which is cemented by our beliefs and tying them all together.

However, even though our nerves fire in certain ways that seem to point to our identity, the I doesn't live in the brain.

Exercise: Where Are You?

Try this exercise right now.

- Close your eyes and take a few deep breaths. Relax fully.

- Contemplate the following: Spatially speaking, where is your sense of I at this moment? Are you in your liver? Colon? Kidneys? It is very easy to understand that of course we are not located in our abdominal organs. Can you be in the brain then? Think of Einstein's preserved brain. Is *he* in his brain? If we dissected your brain, will we find you in there? Think of people that lose limbs in tragic accidents or those that have parts of their brains surgically removed. Do they lose a part of their I?

- If you're not in your body, where are you? If you said mind, you'd be partially correct, but then where is your mind if it is not within your brain cells?

- The popular way of thinking is that the brain creates your I, but we have seen earlier that the body has no capacity to spin stories. Even though our bodies are supremely intelligent, as we shall see later, they act and react by way of chemical and electrical signals. If we performed a laboratory experiment to re-create these signals between nerve and gland cells, would a mind appear? If so, where would it show up?

- If you don't know where you are, can you know who you are? Sure, your body is sitting (or standing or lying down) as you read this, but who are you really?

Notice that when you refer to your body parts, you use prepositions like "mine" that denote they belong to you. Even in daily language, you are assuming that there is an I that owns the body and the mind. Your day-to-day language gives away the fact that you don't really think that you are your body or your mind.

Even though we don't really think we are our body-mind, we continue to identify deeply with it, which causes us to maintain our learned behaviors and fixed ways of thinking and feeling. Patterns of thinking and feeling create specific neurohormonal superhighways, ensuring that we continue to think and act in the same habitual ways. Like hamsters on wheels, we get stuck in our body-mind-I loops. If the body suffers, I suffer. If the mind is shaken up, I become discombobulated. The I is essentially based on fear of suffering and desperate wanting to be free of fear and suffering. And because this cannot be guaranteed, the fragile I fights to keep itself alive.

An ancient definition of health includes being saturated with bliss. We cannot be saturated with bliss if our sense of I is being constantly threatened! The path to bliss requires us to question the very basis of our existence, which we will do when we examine the bliss model in detail in the next chapter.

Summary

- Most of our neurohormonal superhighways are formed before age seven and fortified during adolescence.

- Even though our superhighways have been laid out from our repetitive behavior over the years, it is indeed possible to change their courses. This remarkable ability of the brain to change is known as neuroplasticity.

- Epigenetic studies show us that our neurohormonal superhighways influence our lifestyles, which in turn influence the behavior of our genes. Rebuilding our neuronal superhighways has a direct effect on our genes.

- The default mode network (DMN) is a network of various brain centers that light up simultaneously when focused attention is not required and consists of ruminating over the stories that make up who we think we are.

- Changing our neurohormonal superhighways ends the war with ourselves and with what is.

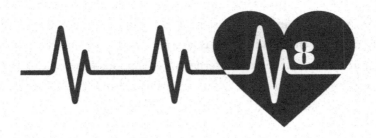

The Bliss Model

As we have seen earlier, studies in psychoneuroimmunology and quantum physics suggest a deep connection between the cosmos and our bodies. Like a hologram, each of us is a perfect replica of the cosmos, carrying within us all the information necessary for healing. In fact, each cell in our bodies reflects the entirety of the cosmos, along with its intelligence. All we need to do is tap into it—"it" being the principle that upholds all of creation.

Ancient sages were immensely gifted seers who discovered the intricate workings of the cosmos and the body, finding that the latter is indeed a holographic image of the former. As they went into deep meditative states, they unraveled these mysteries and passed on the knowledge through a long-preserved verbal tradition. Eventually, their vast knowledge was compiled into various scriptures and texts that became the basis for the study of life, medicine, mind, arts, and so on.

The most significant discovery of the ancient sages was the discovery of the "it" that powers the macrocosm and the microcosm. They found that the "it" is eternal, blissful, and conscious. Eternal bliss consciousness is the fundamental principle out of which the cosmos is born.

While the default model assumes that consciousness arises out of matter (the brain, for instance), the bliss model is based on the premise that matter arose out of bliss consciousness. Not only does bliss give birth to matter, it also becomes it. It is the substance of every animate and inanimate object in the universe. Thus, eternal bliss consciousness is who we really are. When we discover eternal bliss consciousness as our true identity, we gain access to deep healing and freedom from suffering. How does bliss become matter? Let's start at the very beginning.

Bliss Becomes Matter

Bliss consciousness is eternal and rests as a vast potential. Creation begins when consciousness becomes aware of itself. This self-awareness is the first throb of activity in the vast potential (such as the big bang), which expands into infinity to create space and time.

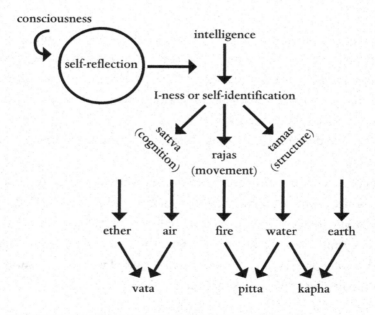

Figure 1: Bliss Consciousness Diagram. Bliss consciousness becomes matter, beginning with the self-referencing throb that is infused with intelligence and self-identification ("I"). Self-identification occurs through sattva, rajas, and tamas—the three qualities (gunas) that differentiate into the five elements of ether, air, fire, water, and earth. The elements combine in specific ways to become vata, pitta, and kapha (doshas), the puppeteers of the cosmos and the body-mind.

The self-awareness gives rise to cosmic "I-ness." This I-ness is the intelligence that knows itself by its three fundamental qualities, known as gunas, which determine the structure and function of the universe. Tamas gives matter its physical structure, rajas provides nature with movement and dynamism, and sattva grants it intelligence. Tamas is heavy and has the quality of inertia; rajas is quick, active, and volatile; and sattva is pure, calm, and sweet.

The throb of self-awareness evolves in loops of ecstatic vibrations forming the five great elements. With each subsequent loop, the vibrations become denser to form ether, air, fire, water, and earth. From the subtle vibrations of the cosmic self-awareness arises the first element, space, or ether. The arising of movement within space gives rise to air. Friction produced by the movement of air gives rise to heat; when particles of heat interact, they combust into the next element, fire. The heat of fire liquefies subtle elements in space, forming water, while solidification of elements in water gives rise to earth. Along with a change in vibration, each element acquires its own unique characteristic of spaciousness, lightness, heat, wetness, and heaviness, these qualities being the result of their differing vibratory frequencies. Quantum physicists agree with the ancient sages that matter is energy, and energy is vibration.

The elements absorb the three qualities of the self-referencing throb. Space, the subtlest of elements, is mainly sattva. Air is predominantly rajas because of its movement, but because of its lightness, it also has sattva. Fire is dynamic, moves quickly, and has rajas; because of its ability to burn everything into uniform ashes without attachment, it also has sattva. Water is also heavy and therefore has tamas; due to its property of flow and movement, it has rajas; and because of its clarity and ability to reflect, it has sattva. Earth is heavy and mainly tamas.

From stars and planets to inanimate substances to us, everything in creation is a combination of the five elements with their corresponding qualities and is governed by awareness. Self-awareness infused with supreme intelligence is responsible for the functioning of the cosmos and controls all natural laws such as gravity, magnetism, force, and velocity. It also drives the functioning of every cellular and sub-cellular structure. It is the force that stimulates a single fertilized cell to divide and differentiate into various types of cells, tissues, organs and organ systems. This intelligence is the reason why stomach cells secrete acid, while bone cells use calcium and heart cells stretch and contract to help pump blood. However, this intelligence is non-personal—as in it doesn't belong to the "I" that we identify with. For instance, digestion, which is the breakdown of ingested food into nutrients and energy, occurs similarly in all organisms; only the details differ based on the species.

Bliss Becomes I

As we saw in chapter 7, my I is made up of all the things I like or dislike as well as the labels that I think make up who I am (big nose, not too smart, good cook, hate meat, and so on). Picked up in early life from our caregivers, we adopt these labels as our own, and the default mode network keeps the story of the I going. Repeated activation of the neurohormonal pathways reinforce the likes and dislikes that form the I story. My I feels very different and unique compared to other ones based on their likes and dislikes that arise from their life experiences. My ability to control some of my body movements, such as speech, hands, and legs, further cements my I, along with my unique human ability to say that I am aware. Where does this I come from?

Like everything else in the cosmos, the I is also powered by the intelligence of the self-aware throb. Bliss powers each one of our trillions of cells to do their immensely complex work of exchanging information, adapting to the environment, responding to stimuli, digesting food and data, and keeping us alive. This intelligence descends in a top-down fashion into the fetus in early pregnancy, corresponding with the development of the heartbeat. Entering through the soft part of the skull, bliss descends down the spine, creating millions of pathways that carry its energetic currents to every cell.

When a baby is born, she does not see herself as separate from her mother and lacks the sense of I. As she approaches her second birthday, she begins to learn about her separateness from those around her. She learns her name, what she's good at, what she must do, and where she belongs, and with this she begins to assert herself with "mine" and "me." This is why this stage is known as the "terrible twos." Bliss that had descended down the spine and until then had been unobscured begins to become veiled by the rapidly forming superhighways that form the story of the I. Although bliss powers the whole process, it becomes ignorant of its own nature. This is like an actor who gets so in character that he forgets who he really is.

In the "Where am I?" exercise in the previous chapter, we came to see that the I doesn't reside anywhere in the physical body, including the brain. We discovered that we will not find you in your brain cells either. So where exactly does this identity reside?

The Three Bodies Powered by Bliss

According to the bliss model, we have not one but three bodies that determine our particular body-mind traits. The physical body is sustained by food. Everything we consume is digested and assimilated into the trillions of cells forming the various organ systems, as we will see in chapter 9.

The subtle body is made up of energy, mind, and intellect. This is where the sense organs and organs of action are registered—the external world is brought in through the sense organs (eyes, nose, ears, tongue, and skin), and our response is sent out through the organs of action (hands for working, tongue for speaking, legs for walking, anus and urethra for excreting, and sex organs for reproducing). The subtle body is made up of the countless channels that run throughout the body and carry prana, the intelligent life force that powers the body and the mind. These channels converge at various points throughout the body, forming chakras (wheels of blissful energy).

Of the millions of unseen channels that crisscross the subtle body, three are most important and run parallel to the spine and look remarkably like the caduceus, the symbol of medicine.

The central channel (sushumna) forms the staff of the caduceus and runs in the center of the spine from the perineum to the top of the head. Running along this staff are the "hot" and "cold" channels (pingala and ida) that periodically wrap around to the other side and correspond to the

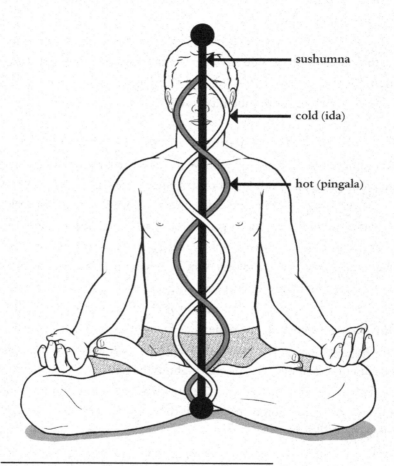

Figure 2: Three Main Channels. The three main channels in the subtle body run along the spine. The central channel, the sushumna, runs in the center of the spine from the perineum to the top of the head, and the "hot" and "cold" channels lie on the sides, periodically wrapping around to the other side. The side channels correspond to the sympathetic and parasympathetic nervous system.

sympathetic and parasympathetic nervous system. However, while the sympathetic and parasympathetic systems power opposite functions of the body, the hot and cold channels fuel the dualistic tendencies of the mind, such as pain/pleasure and likes/dislikes.

Ordinarily, prana switches between the hot and cold channels several times over the course of the day. This periodic switching is the hallmark of the dualistic tendencies of the ordinary mind, marked by constant vacillation between likes and dislikes and the attraction and aversion related to the push and pull of sense objects. As prana switches between the hot and cold channels, it briefly enters the central staff when the breath is even between the nostrils and the mind is quiet. This is easily observed with the breath.

Exercise: **Become Aware of Your Breath**

Try this at various times during the day.

- Place your index finger horizontally under your nostrils and breathe normally. You will notice that the breath is prominent in one nostril. Make note of what you are doing and how you are feeling.

- Notice which nostril is prominent when you wake up or when you're hungry, agitated, peaceful, tired, or sleepy.

- There will be times when the breath is perfectly even in both nostrils. What is your state of mind when this happens?

The subtle body powers the physical body and is in turn fed by the causal body. The causal body is made of impressions and drives the physical and subtle bodies as actions, choices, and thoughts. Impressions are the likes and dislikes that are facilitated by the limbic system and make up the labels and beliefs of the I, which veil the bliss of our true nature. As we have seen, these impressions are formed from past experiences and lock us into habitual thoughts and actions. They bridge our long-gone pasts with our nonexistent futures and keep us in a constant state of war with what is. Without conscious work, impressions turn us into helpless victims of our pasts, our culture, our upbringing and circumstances. They keep us bound in linearity and suffering. The type of impressions we have and how they will affect the quality of our lives is determined by our gunas.

Gunas and the Three Bodies

Recall that arising from the cosmic self-referencing throb of awareness, the three gunas (qualities) make up the basis of all of creation. On the level of the individual, gunas arise from the impressions of the causal body and determine the quality of our minds, bodies, lives, and experiences.

Just as gunas in particular combinations make up the elements that in turn make up all matter, gunas in particular combinations make up our individual psyche, nature, or personality. When tamas is predominant, we are slothful and plagued by inertia, darkness, and lack of motivation. When rajas is predominant, we are driven by determination, ambition, activity (and hyperactivity), anxiety, and restlessness. When sattva is predominant, we experience a quiet mind, clarity, and qualities of sweetness and contentment (see table 1). As we will see in chapter 11, the higher the level of sattva in our psyche, the greater is our ability to know the bliss within.

Tamas	Rajas	Sattva
• Dullness, laziness	• Action and drive, movement, stimulation of the senses and emotions	• Calmness and contentment
• Fatalistic, judgmental, jealous, dark, and depressed	• Anger, over-reactivity, inability to control emotions	• Inherently virtuous, loving, joyful, kind, and giving
• Blame others and the world for our problems	• Dependence on stimulation	• Lack of dependence on outside influence for happiness
• Rigid in beliefs, creating isolation and dissociation from others	• Continual seeking of satisfaction in actions and through senses	• Greater ability to tap into inner bliss

Table 1: The Action of the Gunas in Our Psyche

At this point we might begin to wonder what the gunas or elements have to do with health or disease. Sam's story may be illustrative. He was 58 when he came to see me. He had recently undergone open-heart surgery for coronary artery disease (see chapter 3) with four bypass grafts at another hospital, and was seeking a new cardiologist. At the first visit I noticed that Sam was quiet and withdrawn, talking only when spoken to and answering in monosyllables. It was as if he was so self-absorbed that he had difficulty engaging with anyone else. He would not meet my eyes when he responded to my queries about his health and habits. His wife, who accompanied him, did most of the talking. I adjusted his medications and tried to discuss lifestyle changes, including diet and exercise. I suggested that he walk for about a half hour every day and incorporate more fresh produce in his diet. He nodded his assent, mumbling that he would "try."

When I saw him again in two months, he was not having heart symptoms and was taking his medications. Nothing else had changed. He continued to avert my eyes, remaining self-absorbed. He missed two appointments and returned a year later. Once again, nothing had changed. I could sense his inertia; his wife was trying to get him to change his habits, but he was simply unable to take the first step.

A month later Sam came to the emergency room with a minor heart attack requiring urgent angioplasty of one of the bypass grafts. He came back to my office a week after the hospitalization. This time he was worried and anxious. For the first time since I'd known him, he engaged with me in conversation, asking what he could do to prevent another heart attack. We talked about diet and exercise again. This time he was listening. He asked pointed questions about what he could eat, what he must avoid, what type of exercise he must engage in and how much. I gave him (and his wife) detailed guidelines and resources for recipes and additional information.

Two months later Sam returned to the office, and I was pleased to see he had lost nearly fifteen pounds. Importantly, he was smiling and showed interest in his surroundings. At this point we talked about his job and his daily habits and stress levels. He revealed that he had chronic stress and anxiety that had weighed him down earlier. Although the changes in diet and taking up an exercise program had helped, now he felt the mental noise more acutely. I taught him a simple mindfulness meditation technique and asked him to practice it twice a day without fail. When I saw him again a few weeks later, Sam seemed like a different man. His gait had changed; he was no longer hunching and staring at the ground as he walked. He greeted the office staff and me with pleasantries. He looked fit, happy, and well on his way to health and bliss.

Sam's initial condition was that of tamas, characterized by inertia, mental fog, indecisiveness, and a general sense of heaviness. It took a heart attack to jar him out of tamas into rajas, punctuated by motivation, dynamism, and activity that propelled him into making lifestyle changes. The meditation brought out his sattva, marked by contentment, goodwill, lightness, and clarity. He continues to demonstrate progressive contentment and sweetness indicative of increasing sattva.

Even though the gunas dominate our lives from one moment to the next, we remain unaware of their influence. Although Sam's condition could be treated with medications alone, his spirit needed more for accelerated evolution. The heart attack was the stimulus his spirit needed to catapult him from tamas to rajas. This forced evolution is quite common when catastrophe forces us from inertia into positive action. I've seen patients change their behaviors overnight and become magnificent advocates for their own care. We are pushed into evolutionary change by the very intelligence that powers us.

Everything in the cosmos is an interaction between the five great elements; however, this is not the full story. The five elements combine further, in specific combinations, into three main principles or energies that go on to create the structure and functioning of the universe, including our body-mind. These principles are called doshas.

Doshas: The Hidden Puppeteers

The three doshas arising from the five elements make up the unique fingerprint of our body-mind. Vata arises from the combination of ether and air and is the principle of movement that regulates all moving activities in the body, such as breathing and the passage of food through the digestive tract, blood through the heart and arteries, and micronutrients through cellular membranes. It also regulates the movement of thought and emotions and all changes in our lives. Movement is the hallmark of existence, while stillness is that of death. For this reason, vata is called the king dosha.

Fire and water mingle to form pitta, the principle of heat and transformation. Pitta regulates metabolism and digestion. Pitta is the energy of the digestive enzymes that break down food to nutrients and waste, the processing of nutrients at the cellular level, and the transformation of one thing (for example, food) to another (nutrients and waste). It is the force of every one of the billions of chemical reactions that are responsible for maintaining the precise workings of the body. Pitta is the principle that digests and processes thoughts, emotions, sense perceptions (taste, smell, sight, sound, and touch), and life experiences. Without pitta, we would have no ability to learn from our experiences or make sense of our moment-to-moment interactions with the world.

Water and earth combine to form kapha, the principle of structure. Kapha regulates the structure of cells, tissues, and organs and maintains the proportions of water within various bodily structures, being responsible for the lubrication of joints, secretions of all cellular structures, and retention of fluid where it is needed.

Doshas are the animators of life. Consider the difference between a live and dead body. At one point in time, a body is a beloved parent, friend, or family member. At another, it is a dead body that needs to be disposed of within a certain period. Along with grief, we may experience fear, disgust, or unease with the body. If we think deeply, a loved one we couldn't part with becomes a body we can't wait to dispose of when it is bereft of the doshas that translate into life. With the loss of vata, the breath, heart, digestion, brain pathways, and mind functioning come to an end. Loss of pitta decreases the body temperature, and metabolism ceases. Withdrawal of kapha dries up tissues with loss of structural integrity. Doshas are the master puppeteers of the body-mind. Through their functions, they animate a body and turn it into a desirable being. When they are withdrawn, the body loses its attractiveness and becomes an inanimate object.

In the default model we separate the workings of the body from that of the mind, and in this linear logic we can see no connection between heartburn and anger. In the bliss model, on the other hand, the trees and the forest are seen as a whole. Thus, we understand that when pitta becomes aggravated, it not only causes an overproduction of stomach acid, causing reflux and heartburn, but its heating action on the mind also causes anger and aggression.

Specific combinations of doshas are determined at conception and dictate our distinctive body frame, facial features, and fingerprints. Specific dosha combinations determine our susceptibility to problems in specific organ systems. Since doshas are made up of elements that have gunas embedded in them, they also drive the peculiar ways in which we think and feel.

As long as the unique proportions of the three doshas that make up your body remain stable, you will remain free of disease. In this model balance isn't about getting all three doshas in equal proportions (unless, of course, that is your particular constitution), but it is about getting you back to your own unique state of balance. When it comes to the mind, however, the goal of this model is to cultivate sattva, which enables the spilling over of your inner bliss into your body, leading to healing and beauty. Importantly, this type of healing leads to the end of rebirth into suffering.

Rebirth into Suffering

Have you wondered how children turn out to be prodigies? Consider Mozart, who started composing at age five, when most children are yet to learn the basics of music. How did he acquire the depth of knowledge required for musical composition at such a tender age? One theory that explains such phenomena is that of reincarnation.

According to this theory, the causal and subtle layers exit the physical body at the time of death, and depending upon the type of impressions and desires that need to be expressed and fulfilled, they find a host for the next birth. The theory has it that we select the parents, culture, and community who will pass on genetic traits and lifestyle habits that will help us express the desires we have accumulated in the previous birth. Our causal body then starts directing our choices and actions with the determined purpose of fulfilling particular desires. If your strongest desire is to express musical ability picked up in an earlier birth, you will be born in a family of musicians with the resources to fulfill a musical career.

This theory also explains why children born of the same parents and raised in the same family differ in their personalities. Our unique personalities—with idiosyncrasies, preferences, aversions, and talents—are products not only of the impressions of this lifetime, but also of the previous ones. The issue is that even as we fulfill old desires, we keep accumulating new ones because of the neurohormonal superhighways we build through seeking things to make us happy. Thus, we are born again and again in an endless cycle.

However, the theory of reincarnation is of no practical use in daily life. It is not necessary to believe in reincarnation to see how we are reborn into suffering. We simply have to look at the human predicament that leads to desire. When we have what we desire, we become attached to it and fear losing it. When we don't get what we desire, it consumes us with restlessness. What we desire is based on our past experiences that we project into the future. For instance, if success brought me temporary pleasure in the past, I seek more of it, thinking I will be happy in the future when I am more successful. All of my choices and actions are determined by the emotional impression of desire, where we characterize all experience into good and bad, want and don't want, like and dislike. As we give in to the impression in our thoughts and actions, we create deep grooves of habit. The impression and the habit start to feel like the I, our identity.

The unique predicament of the I is that it craves completion and contentment. In the default model we think the I is our body-mind and innocently believe that our happiness comes from external objects. Thus, we are driven to desperately seek them. For example, if you are the sort that likes cars, you may covet a particular model. As long as you don't have the car, the desire for it defines who you are by creating the turmoil of wanting. You're filled with bliss the moment you procure the car. You mistakenly think that acquiring the car made you happy, when in reality your bliss is the result of the temporary end of wanting.

Desire: The Fuel of Suffering

Desire is the fuel of the I, and when a particular desire is fulfilled, the I temporarily loses fuel and dies. For a brief moment you gain access to our inherent bliss, which was previously obscured by the turmoil of desire. However, the dopamine-seeking pathways soon become reactivated. Your eye catches a better-looking car with state-of-the-art features. The nagging of desire is stirred up, and the I is reborn. As long as the I seeks completion from external objects, it is bound to suffer. You may not have the resources to get that new model. Even if you did, you see that there is always something that is better out there. You suffer because the permanent happiness you seek never comes. The I reincarnates again and again into suffering.

Our habitual patterns are so deeply ingrained in the causal and subtle bodies that we seem to be propelled along by their sheer power, being reborn again and again into suffering. Like a hamster on a wheel, we run along the well-worn grooves, helplessly reacting in the same old ways to everything that arises in our experience.

For true healing to occur and to get off the cycle of rebirth into suffering, we must become willing to change our habitual ways at any cost. This is how we return to bliss.

Returning to Bliss

A "dis-ease" is an accurate signal that our current patterns of thoughts, emotions, and behaviors are not serving us—we are not at ease. If we change how we view disease, everything about it changes—our relationship with it, our response to treatment, and that elusive thing, healing.

The purport of healing holistically is to find and work on the root cause of an ailment. Thus, working on the body alone does not result in healing—it results in "treatment," a word with a different connotation, which is the use of agents like drugs or surgery in an attempt to cure or mitigate a disease. Working on the subtle body alone does not work either since it doesn't get to the root of the issue. For true healing to occur, we need to work on the causal body, which consists of the conglomeration of beliefs that make up the I.

As consciousness descends into matter and forms the body-mind, it becomes obscured by the preoccupations of the mind and obsession with the body. For us to return to the bliss of our true nature, the ideal body-mind state is one of balance. When the body returns to balance and the mind rests in sattva, we remember that our true nature is pure bliss consciousness. Once accessed, this bliss pervades our senses, bodies, and minds, and we discover beauty, love, and harmony in our daily lives. We return to health.

The path to balance and bliss leads to an overhaul of our bodies and minds. In the next chapter we will see how to ignite the power of transformation that takes us from rebirth into suffering to permanent bliss.

Summary

- Each of us is a perfect replica of the cosmos. Within us we carry all the information necessary for healing.

- Bliss consciousness is the substance of every animate and inanimate object in the universe. It is who we really are.

- Bliss consciousness evolves into the five great elements: ether, air, fire, water, and earth, which form the basis of everything in creation.

- According to the bliss model, we have not one but three bodies that determine our particular body-mind traits.

- The physical body is sustained by food; the subtle body is made up of energy, mind, and intellect; and the causal body is made of the impressions of who we think we are—the I that veils the bliss of our true nature.

- Gunas (qualities) in particular combinations make up our individual psyche, nature, or personality. Tamas leads to inertia, laziness, and darkness; rajas to determination, ambition, anxiety, and restlessness; and sattva to a quiet mind, clarity, sweetness, and contentment. The higher the sattva in our psyche, the greater is our ability to see the bliss within.

- The three doshas (principles) arising from the five elements make up the unique fingerprint of our body-mind. Vata is the principle of movement, pitta is the principle of transformation, and kapha is the principle of structure.

- Desire is the fuel of the I. When a particular desire is fulfilled, the I temporarily loses fuel and dies, which reveals the bliss of our true nature—until desires are stirred up again. Since there is no way for all our desires to be fulfilled, the I reincarnates again and again into suffering.

- The ideal condition for us to remember the bliss of our true nature is for the body to return to balance and our mind to rest in sattva.

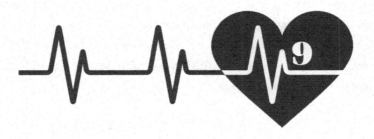

The Fire of Life

The path from suffering to bliss is one of radical transformation. In Ayurveda this transformation is facilitated by what is known as the inner fire. In this chapter we will explore what this inner fire is, how it acts in our body-minds, and how its imbalance affects us. Balancing our inner fire is an integral part of the Bliss Rx.

Fire is a significant component of worship and rituals in many cultures. Fire rituals were performed in ancient times to attain specific results, such as rain in times of drought or relief from plague or other contagions. The deity of the desired outcome (for example, rain) was propitiated through the element of fire via offerings of grain, fruit, fragrant wood or incense, ghee (clarified butter), and other ingredients into a specially constructed fire pit. As the fire burned, mantras (words, phrases, or prayer) were chanted to absorb the fire's energies. It was believed that fire had the power to carry the prayers and aspirations of humans to celestial realms, then carry divine blessings back to humans.

Known as agni, this inner fire plays the central role in our physiology. It is the fire that maintains life, preserves the functions of the body, and determines whether we are afflicted with disease and how we think and feel. It is often associated only with digestion, but not of food alone. Agni is the intermediary between our external and internal worlds. It enables us to take in the world through our senses, process it on the physical, subtle, and causal levels, and act accordingly. It is the pulse of intelligence within each cell, organ, and organ system, as well as the mind, intellect, and emotion. Impaired or dysfunctional agni is therefore the root of all ailments of the mind and body.

Agni: The Force for Transformation

On the physical level, agni aids digestion of food through the marvelous cascade of digestive enzymes and juices produced in the mouth (saliva), stomach (gastric juice), and intestines (bile and pancreatic juices) that progressively break down food into smaller and smaller components that can finally be carried by the circulatory system to every cell of the body. Pause for a moment and consider this. The oatmeal you had for breakfast this morning is steadily being transformed into your cells! Your body is not only sustained by food, but at the most basic level is the result of the magical transformation of food into what you see in the mirror. Agni is what makes this transformation possible through the intelligent cascade of enzymes, hormones, and chemicals. Just as the heat of cooking makes food more digestible or palatable, the heat of agni in the various chemical reactions enables the conversion of what we consume to the structure of the body.

At the cellular level, agni takes the form of the principle that governs the actions of the subcellular structures and the pathways of cellular metabolism, converting the gross components of nutrients to their subtle essences of prana (energy), tejas (radiance), and ojas (immunity). Prana, tejas, and ojas are the subtle purified essences of the three doshas, which determine the functioning of the body and the mind.

Prana

Prana (called chi by the Chinese and mana by the Polynesians) is energy, the subtle essence of the vata dosha. If you've ever been in a yoga class, you've probably heard the instructor asking you to breathe in certain ways to increase prana in your body. You may have felt a freshness, aliveness, vibrancy, or a sensation of tingling during certain breath exercises or in other situations like being in nature. Although prana is most often associated with the breath, it is not the breath. It is the life force that makes breathing (as well as all other body functions) possible. When prana is depleted, life comes to an end. As we saw in chapter 8, prana resides in the subtle body, flowing through thousands of invisible channels that crisscross throughout the body and supply every cell. When prana flows evenly through these channels, the body is adequately nourished and displays vitality and absence of disease.

Prana is responsible for growth, how we adapt to our changing situations, and equilibrium of the body and the mind. It promotes healing via the immune system and enables the movement of electrical impulses from one neuron to the next in the nervous system. Prana is the life-creating force of our reproductive system and therefore determines how long we live and the quality of our lives. Evenness of prana corresponds to evenness of the mind and fuels creativity and enthusiasm for an activity. Erratic flow of prana results in hyperactivity of the mind, lack of clarity and concentration, anxiety, and misapprehension.

The amount and quality of our prana is determined by the quality of our agni. Agni finds and soaks up the essence of the air we breathe, the food we eat, and the water we drink, converting it to prana and propelling it through its innumerable channels.

Tejas

Tejas is inner radiance, the subtle essence of the pitta dosha. It is the quality of light and heat within us that enables the "cooking" of food into its various nutrients and of sensory perceptions, thoughts, and impressions. Consider this: How does your brain process a Granny Smith apple? It only sees "green" and "round," and it has no ability to call it an apple or the feeling it evokes in you. Tejas is the principle that converts the brain's information into the meaningful sensory perception of "Yummy! A juicy apple!" and of the associated action of your hand reaching for it.

Tejas drives the hormonal system (particularly the thyroid, pancreas, and adrenal glands), maintains body temperature, and gives skin its luster and coloration. Since it controls metabolic processes, imbalanced tejas leads to imbalances in electrolytes (such as sodium, magnesium, and others) in the blood. In the immune system, tejas is the force that enables the recognition and destruction of toxins and microbes. Most importantly, a derangement in tejas is the root cause of all inflammatory conditions in the body, including heart disease, arthritis, cancer, and others; more on this later.

In the mind, tejas is responsible for our determination and drives us to purposeful action. It is quite literally "the fire in the belly" that spurs us on our chosen path. An out-of-balance tejas leads to greed, excessive competitiveness, insatiable ambition, anger, hostility, and vindictiveness on one extreme, and lack of drive, laziness, and inertia on the other.

Tejas is the heat of prana and is assimilated into the body and mind by agni. Think of the flames of a fire in your fireplace. Prana is like the height of the flames, while tejas is the associated heat. Agni is the amount and quality of oxygen in the air that fans the fire. The more balanced the agni, the more even the prana and the tejas.

Ojas

Ojas is the vital reserve of the body and the subtle essence of the kapha dosha. It is the end result of balanced agni and the digestive process that results in immunity, strength, and endurance. You can't miss someone with abundant ojas—they are filled with optimism, youthfulness, seemingly endless stamina, and the ability to accomplish many tasks with unearthly ease. When we think of digestion, we may only think of the stomach and intestines. However, digestion in Ayurveda is said to be an elaborate process that progresses through the various tissues and takes nearly a month for completion.

Digestion begins in the stomach and the intestines, where nutrients are absorbed and waste products are excreted. The absorbed nutrients are carried to the liver, where agni breaks them down into their fundamental molecular elements, forming the following in succession: plasma, blood, muscle, fat, bone, nerves, and, finally, reproductive tissue. Each tissue has its own agni, which takes in the material from the previous tissue and turns it into what it needs. At each stage of tissue formation, increasingly subtle wastes are removed from the body. Ojas is the final product of this elaborate process. Milky and ephemeral, it is said that a healthy body has a single handful of ojas: five drops of this reside in the heart.

Ojas is the crux of our immune, nervous, and reproductive systems. It is the subtle essence that lines the cells, giving them structure and enabling the flow of prana. The strength and quality of agni determines the amount and quality of ojas. In the previous example of the flame, ojas determines the strength of the flame and how long it will last.

The quality of our ojas determines how we respond to stress and change. When our ojas is depleted, we become overwhelmed, lose our sense of humor, and feel like we have lost direction. An imbalance in any one of the three subtle essences results in an imbalance in the other two. Conversely, the effort to improve the quality of any one of them results in improvement in the other two.

Imbalanced Agni

Pause for a moment and reflect on the image of a fire in the fireplace. When you picture it in your mind's eye, what is its most predominant quality? It is a source of light and heat, of course, but if there is one word you could describe it with, what would it be? The word that pops up in my mind is dynamic. It does not remain still and is constantly changing form, turning fuel into ash.

Picture the following scenario. You are out camping with your friends on a beautiful summer evening. Someone decides that a campfire is in order, and you take charge of building it. If you were a Scout, as I was, you have this down pat. You choose the ideal spot based on the direction of the wind and the elevation of the ground and away from dead bush. Next, you start gathering the required materials: tinder to start the fire such as dry leaves, kindling such as small branches to get the fire going, and fuel wood such as bigger logs and branches to keep the fire burning.

The campfire is the analogy for agni, while some of the common issues with building it represent the issues that lead to its dysfunction in the body-mind. If you decide to build the fire on a day when there are gusts of wind, the strength of your fire will vary. The flames rise and subside with the wind. Inconsistency of agni in the body-mind leads to inconsistent digestion. If you have this type of digestive power, your agni will be variable, and if I were to ask you about hunger, bowel movements, sleep, or state of mind, you might answer that they are inconsistent; you are hungry some days but not others, you are constipated some of the time but not always, you sleep well some nights but toss and turn on others, you catch your mind racing some days but not always. This variable agni is the hallmark of an imbalance in vata.

Going back to the imagery of the campfire, if you decide to build it on dry grass in an area with an overgrowth of dry underbrush, you will quickly have a disaster on your hands as the fire spreads uncontrollably. This is what happens when the agni is overactive. If this is your condition, you might respond to the above questions differently. You might be so hungry before a meal that you see red! You might have frequent diarrhea and heartburn, get easily upset and angry in interactions, and have a hard time going to sleep. Overactive agni is the sign of pitta imbalance.

Now imagine that you've built the campfire in a safe place and have successfully started it with tinder and kindling. What would happen if I placed a bundle of large, wet logs as the fire began? They would choke the flames, analogous of an underactive agni. You'd recognize this to be your condition if you never felt hungry, if you frequently felt like the food you ate just sat for hours in your stomach, if you were more often constipated than not, felt unrefreshed upon waking up even when you feel you've had a good night's sleep, and often felt unmotivated and lazy. An underactive agni is the sign of kapha imbalance.

If your campfire was built under ideal conditions where the flame remains steady and the byproduct is a uniform ash, that would correspond to a balanced agni, where the various tissues undergo appropriate metabolism and excrete the unwanted byproducts; the mind is filled with sweetness, contentment, enthusiasm for life, and love for self and others; and the senses are pervaded by bliss.

Recall that the essential quality of agni is dynamism. An imbalance in agni therefore results in the opposing quality of stagnation. This quality of stagnation is called ama. Ama is the subtle substance that is responsible for the many physical, mental, and emotional manifestations of imbalanced agni.

Ama, Disease, and Suffering

When agni is out of balance, digestion and metabolism in the body and mind suffer. Not only is there incomplete digestion of food in the stomach and intestines, but also at the subsequent tissue levels. Ordinarily, unique waste products are eliminated at each step of tissue metabolism. However, a variable hyperactive or underactive agni is unable to complete the metabolic process. The residue is a subtle substance that is the opposite of ojas. Instead of the sweet-smelling, milky, and nourishing ojas that lines cellular membranes in the state of balanced agni, what accumulates is the sticky, foul-smelling, and heavy ama. The digestive tract is the first place where the ama accumulates, presenting as diarrhea, heartburn, sticky stools, indigestion, loss of taste and appetite, and abnormal weight gain. When it goes unrecognized, ama begins to disseminate from the digestive tract into the deeper tissues, accumulating between cells and clogging the channels of the organ systems.

At the physical level, ama deposition in cellular membranes and in between cells results in disruption of tissue metabolism. In arteries ama accumulation causes a disruption in the endothelial lining, and inflammation ensues. Similarly, disruption of channels of elimination leads to stiffness and degeneration in joints; fibromyalgia, fatigue, and pain in muscles; fat accumulation leading to metabolic syndrome, diabetes, high blood pressure, high cholesterol, and obesity; menstrual disorders such as heavy periods with clotting and pain; fibrocystic changes in breasts and ovaries; symptoms of congestion such as chronic sinus pain, swelling, and water accumulation; post-nasal drip; and skin disorders such as acne and other blemishes. As ama continues to accumulate in particular channels, cellular immunity diminishes and can result in autoimmune diseases as well as various cancers.

The particular channels that become clogged and result in particular diseases and conditions depend upon the specific weaknesses of our body-minds, based on the superhighways we have built in our brains, the habits and lifestyles we have accrued, and the genes we have inherited (remember, however, that the latter is minor compared to our habits and lifestyles).

At the subtle level, ama leads to the tamasic state of inertia, laziness, dark moods, greed, cunning, hatred, sloppiness, and an overall distorted perception of life or the rajasic state of mental and physical hyperactivity, inability to sit still, lack of concentration, aggression, competitiveness, rivalry, hostility, anger, outbursts of rage and violence, and lack of regard for others. Quite simply, ama obscures bliss and health.

At the causal level, ama traps us further into suffering and takes us further away from bliss. A balanced agni leads to the sattvic state of bliss characterized by contentment, mental quiet, peace, happiness, equanimity, and compassion.

However, as important as ama is as a causative factor for disease, it is not to blame in many instances where disease occurs merely as an imbalance of doshas even in the absence of ama. Imbalance of doshas is also mediated by agni.

Fire, Mind, and Heart

As we begin to understand agni, we learn to decipher our relationship with food, exercise, and other lifestyle choices. For instance, if we are unable to digest and release past trauma and pain, food becomes the comforting factor used to cover up the underlying discomfort. Eventually, food turns into the enslaving master of our senses and our lives, resulting in obesity and disease. In this case, the imbalance of agni that makes it difficult to process our past events is the root cause of our food addiction. We can go on diets, undergo bariatric surgery, restrict calories or food groups through mental dialogue, or exercise obsessively to lose weight.

Focusing entirely on the body, we can push away the pain and try to forget that it is there.

However, the imbalance of agni continues unchecked where the pain lurks in the background, ready to rear its head at the first given opportunity. Sooner or later the pain wins, and the benefits gained through "hard work" dissipate with a vengeance. All the weight returns, and the cycle of suffering goes on endlessly.

When eating to mask deeper issues, food can provide comfort while eating and shortly thereafter, but, like all other substance addictions, it is accompanied by guilt, shame, and inadequacy a few minutes or hours later. The vicious cycle of eating-feeling bad-eating thus propagates itself in a spiral. We are at war with our bodies. Like violent wars in the world, these internal wars can never fulfill our wish for good health or to feel better about ourselves. We assume that it will be easier to accept ourselves after we lose the weight and have our lives together. Such a future time never arrives because the fundamental problem of self-loathing has not been addressed. This is a pattern I see on a daily basis in my medical practice. It is the result of an out-of-balance agni, the mental and emotional effects of which cannot be escaped.

On the other hand, as soon as we begin to accept (and, further, love) ourselves just the way we are, we have set the motion for agni to return to balance. When the fire begins to burn steadily, the courage to deal with our past experiences and current life situations begins to arise magically from deep within. Our neurohormonal superhighways begin to change course, resulting in the transformation of our physical, subtle, and causal bodies. Bringing the agni back to balance is therefore the first step toward healing.

The Fiery Ritual of Bliss

Ultimately, agni is the consciousness that determines whether we cling to suffering or return to our rightful nature of bliss. Symbolic of the rituals of the old days, we can learn to pour our thoughts, emotions, habits, actions and lifestyles into this steady, calm, and benevolent fire. Like the ideally built campfire, agni uses everything we offer to it as fuel and trans-forms it into ojas, the sweet nectar. Ojas is known as the bliss molecule since its quality and quantity are also dependent on those of prana and tejas. Balancing agni to increase the quality and quantity of ojas is there-fore the goal of the Bliss Rx, as we will see in part 2.

Summary

- Agni is the principle that maintains life, preserves the functions of the body, and determines whether we are afflicted with disease and how we think and feel.

- Impaired or dysfunctional agni is the root of all ailments of the mind and body.

- Agni converts the gross components of nutrients to the subtle essences of prana (energy), tejas (radiance), and ojas (immunity), the subtle purified essences of the three doshas that determine the functioning of the body and mind.

- Prana is the subtle essence of vata and is responsible for growth, how we adapt to our changing situations, and equilibrium of the body and mind.

- Tejas is the subtle essence of pitta and controls metabolic processes, determination, and purposeful action.

- Ojas is the subtle essence of kapha that determines immunity, strength, and endurance. The quality of our ojas determines how we respond to stress and change.

- An imbalance in agni results in stagnation, which is called ama. Ama is the subtle substance that is responsible for the many physical, mental, and emotional manifestations of disease.

- A balanced agni enables our neurohormonal superhighways to change course, resulting in transformation of our physical, subtle, and causal bodies. Therefore, the first step toward healing is bringing agni back into balance.

Part 2

The Bliss Rx

Now that we have seen the basis and logic for the default and bliss models, we will delve into the principles and practices of the Bliss Rx that will lead to the wellness outcomes described in chapter 1. We will tread this path in a stepwise fashion, integrating the lessons of each step before moving on to the next. The Bliss Rx encompasses your entire being: your body, mind, spirit, senses, perception, how you view the world and yourself, your habits and lifestyle.

If you apply these principles and diligently practice as prescribed, your entire being will begin to transform and heal. Your body will feel lighter, your perception will become increasingly clearer, and your habits and lifestyle will change in wholesome ways. Let's now see what the Bliss Rx entails.

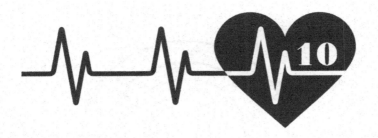

Introduction to
the Bliss Rx

Imagine a rain-fed marsh in the woods on a bright sunny day. The water is thick with silt and debris. Without an outlet, the water stands still and the bright disk of the sun is barely reflected in the dense water. Now think of rapids. In this water the sun is reflected, but its image in the water is choppy and unclear. Next, imagine a mountain lake where the water is calm, still, and serene. The sun is reflected flawlessly, its image in the water indistinguishable from the one in the sky. The sun represents bliss, our true nature. The rain-fed, silty lake represents the state of tamas or inertia, where bliss is completely obscured. The choppy water of the rapids is symbolic of rajas, the state of activity and hyperactivity where bliss is sometimes known and sometimes not, depending on the current. The still mountain lake represents sattva, the state in which bliss can be known directly. With this direct knowledge, suffering comes to an end and healing begins to occur at the primordial and cellular levels.

In this program, we work in an outside-in fashion to work the three bodies that obscure bliss, bringing every aspect of your life back into balance (see figure 3). Balance enables us to return to sattva, like the calm mountain lake where the sun's reflection can be unbroken and untainted.

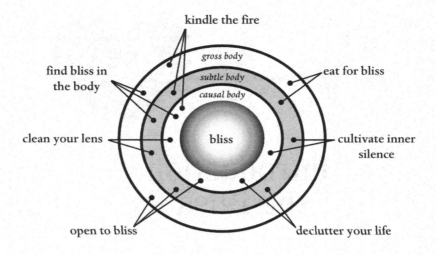

kindle the fire

find bliss in
the body

eat for bliss

clean your lens

bliss

cultivate inner
silence

open to bliss

declutter your life

gross body

subtle body

causal body

Figure 3: Outside In. In the Bliss Rx we work in an outside-in fashion on the
gross, subtle, and causal bodies that obscure the bliss of our true nature.
Each aspect of this prescription works on one or more of the three bodies.

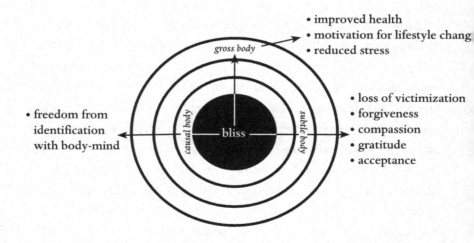

- improved health
- motivation for lifestyle chang
- reduced stress

- loss of victimization
- forgiveness
- compassion
- gratitude
- acceptance

- freedom from
  identification
  with body-mind

gross body

causal body

bliss

subtle body

Figure 4: Inside Out. The result of following the Bliss Rx is the
radiation of the bliss of our true nature outward into the world via
the three bodies, which are transformed into health and well-being
(gross body) and a radical change in perspective (subtle body)
from loss of identification as the body-mind (causal body).

When bliss begins to permeate our senses, our minds, our hearts, and our actions, health is restored in an inside-out fashion (figure 4). When we begin to live our lives as bliss, we change the structure of the cosmos. Yes, each of us is that significant and that powerful.

Every choice, every thought, and every action that occurs daily takes us one step toward or away from bliss and, by default, health. Nothing can be excluded in our pursuit of bliss—the way we brush our teeth, greet our spouse, look in the mirror, talk to the barista, drive our car, relate to others (our children, colleagues, customers or parents), prepare our food, eat our meals, exercise our body, and nurture our mind. Everything counts. It is not just what we do but how we do it that makes a world of difference in whether we are moving closer to sattva or to tamas.

A Word About Timelines

This program is not a quick fix. In my live programs, many people show up for the first session enthusiastic and ready to "get rid of" their pain, stress, blood pressure, or heart disease. When I teach them to meditate, they begin the practice with the mindset of "getting there." When a few find that they are not "getting there" over the next week, they stop the practice.

Think of how long it took you to form the neurohormonal superhighways that drive your daily life. Heart disease is the perfect example of habits acquired over a lifetime culminating in disease. Atherosclerosis begins in childhood and continues to develop and fester over many decades, fostered by ongoing ama and agni imbalance. Heart disease is proof of being on the wheel of our conditioned ways and habits for decades. Undoing those habits takes time. If only we could get off the wheel with one session of meditation! The journey to sattva is highly individual and never ends. Even after we discover bliss to be our true nature, the purification of our bodies and minds continues endlessly. How long does it take to discover bliss? The answer is this: as long as it takes. The journey is the goal. It is critically important to get out of the instant gratification mindset when we come to this, the most significant journey of our lives.

In this program we begin with the end in mind, which is to discover the inherent bliss of our true nature. If followed through, we will find halfway through that the end has magically disappeared. We will find that there is nowhere to get to because we were already always right here, standing as bliss.

The Bliss Rx is for a systematic undoing of our habitual ways of thinking and doing and for recharting our neurohormonal superhighways. It is a steady progression from tamas to rajas to sattva. The basic requirement for this progression is absolute honesty with ourselves. In this program there is nobody to answer to other than ourselves. If we are not completely honest, we run the risk of not making progress and remaining in the states of confusion and inertia.

The entire premise of this prescription is to step out of the grooves of conditioning and habit that keep us from discovering bliss. We do this by replacing nonserving grooves of conditioning (tamasic and rajasic) with wholesome and nurturing ones (sattvic). The process is more about undoing and unlearning than acquiring new skills. Even though you will learn new skills, it is important to know that bliss is what you are already. You will not gain bliss from any skill, program, or teacher. Programs, practices, and teachers can only point you to the truth of your own being.

It can be tempting to tackle the whole program at once. In this case, it can be overwhelming and cause you to give up entirely. It is best to take it one step at a time, moving on to the next as and when you feel comfortable. This is called self-pacing. On the other hand, you will not make much progress if you remain at one step for too long. In general, an adequate period to get adjusted to each step is about three to twelve weeks. It takes twenty-one days of consistent practice to create a new neurohormonal superhighway, whether it is giving up salt or taking up meditation. The key word here is consistent. If you practice one day a week and go about your old ways the rest of the time, the effects are unpredictable and it is much less likely to become a new habit.

Every step is nurturing and nourishing, with an emphasis on favoring one choice over another without undue force. For this, you must want bliss and peace. You must want it more than the choice that presents itself on a moment-to-moment basis. For instance, when you are faced with the choice of waking up early to sit quietly in meditation or stealing a few more minutes of sleep, what you really want will make the choice for you. Mere lip service of wanting to end our suffering will not suffice if we are committed to carrying on with our old ways. Through the course of this program, you will discover, often surprisingly, that your conditioning and habits are so powerful that they often overshadow the desire for bliss, particularly in the beginning. When this happens, you can simply acknowledge their power. Becoming aware of this force is enough to dissolve it. The only thing that gives a habit its power is being completely unaware of it. As soon as we become aware of it as merely a neurohormonal phenomenon, we take away the power we have unconsciously assigned to it.

Our journey to bliss is marked by a few common, distinctive phases. It helps to know of them beforehand so that you are not surprised when you are faced with the characteristic issues of a particular phase.

Common Phases of Evolution

While the phases of progression along the Bliss Rx are laid out as if they are discrete and removed from each other, this is often not the case. You may never experience all the stages, or you may have the insights and symptoms of more than one. There is no particular timeline for each of these stages. Each can last weeks, months, or years, depending upon your unique body-mind makeup. Further, there may be other stages that are not described here and are the result of you exploring uncharted territory! Whatever the case, the following is meant to be a very general guideline and is not set in stone.

Trepidation

In this phase you are not quite sure if you are ready to commit to this program. You may be afflicted with doubt, confusion, or even a sense of dread about what is to come. Some (or all) of what you have read thus far may contradict your beliefs and past learning, causing considerable inner conflict. In the end you eventually decide to give it a try. Even when you begin with the program, you may not be sure if this is for you. As you start seeing some results, no matter how minor, you start to get more comfortable with the program and your commitment strengthens.

Harmony

Once you commit to the program and begin to practice sincerely, the immediate changes in your life are filled with harmony. In this phase your mind begins to settle into quiet and peace. Many people in this stage state that they are experiencing this extent of peace for the first time in their lives. You may feel calmer, sleep better, and experience less anxiety or anger. Your blood pressure may fall, and symptoms such as palpitations or chronic pain may seem less intense. Your commitment continues to strengthen in this phase, when the initial effects very rapidly highlight the difference between stress and peace. The changes are noticeable because they are occurring in your conscious mind.

Stagnation

Since the changes in the previous phase occurred so rapidly, the next phase of stagnation will seem like a drag. Even though you continue with the practices of the program, you may feel that you are not making much progress. You may feel that you are still at peace but there are no additional benefits. In this phase the stillness and peace cultivated through practices are seeping into the subconscious mind and deeper into your body. The changes are occurring more quietly, and, like a storm gathering force, continued practice will result in the next phase of obvious changes.

Turmoil

The purpose of this program is to heal from the inside out. A Band-Aid approach of masking underlying issues does not serve the greater purpose of healing. As the practices take hold, their transformative power begins to stir the subconscious mind, and deep, forgotten hurts from the past surface into conscious awareness. This phase of turmoil can be quite uncomfortable if you happen to go through it but don't understand what is going on. I often call this the "washing machine" phase, where our deep-rooted issues are wrung out of us through the powerful practices of the program. Remember the purpose of the program and know that if you begin to experience irritation, anxiety, sleeplessness, or even physical symptoms like palpitations, you can cut back on practices like meditation and breathing exercises. I will explain this in detail in the related chapters. It is important to continue with the program at this point. If you give up now, you might get stuck in your old, nonserving patterns and feel helpless to make the necessary changes that lead a happier, more fulfilled life.

Stability

The phase of turmoil begins to pass as you continue with the practices and remain steadfast in your path. Often it is only in retrospect that we know the turmoil has passed. It is like suddenly realizing that the nagging headache you've had for the last week is no longer there. Unlike the previous plateau phase of stagnation, this phase of stability gives you a sense of confidence that all is well and that you are making progress. You begin to see that the issues of the past and anxieties of the future have no power over your well-being without your permission. These issues may continue to arise, but you now have honed the tools you've been given and know how to deal with them effectively. You've stuck with the program and are rewarded with the uncovering of your inner fountain of knowledge, joy, and sweetness.

Bliss

As you continue on the program, you will realize that the greatest enemies and wars you can ever face are in your own mind. As this knowledge from the previous phases flowers in you as a living, dynamic reality, you will begin to access the bliss of your true nature. Through the practice of self-inquiry you will come to see that you are not your thoughts, senses, perception, states of consciousness, or body. What you are is beyond description, but if you were to define it, it would be eternal, blissful awareness. As you learn to release the false identification with the body and mind, becoming more established in the bliss of your nature, you will come to realize that everything in your experience is also of the same blissful nature of awareness. You will begin to wake up to oneness with all of existence.

Dealing with the Phases

At any point in the program and at any phase, we can regroup and recommit to changing our destinies when we fall off the course. At all times we remain true to the compass within, which becomes functional as we kindle our agni by following a disciplined routine and dietary guidelines outlined in chapters 11 and 12. We can get back to our inner work through the regular and committed practices of meditation, breath regulation (as in chapters 13 and 15), and our outer lives (through the decluttering practice in chapter 14). We can practice becoming gently vigilant of our inner lives through the self-inquiry practices of chapter 16. As our agni comes into balance and we become more sattvic, we come to experience our bodies in magical ways, facilitated by the exercises in chapter 17. The natural result of this process is the overflowing of bliss to all around us.

The first step in returning to balance in our body-mind is to kindle the fire of digestion, which we will explore in the next chapter.

Summary

- For this program it is critically important to get out of the instant gratification mindset.

- The Bliss Rx is for a systematic undoing of our habitual ways of thinking and doing, and for recharting our neurohormonal superhighways.

- Every step of the program is nurturing and nourishing, with an emphasis on favoring one choice over another without undue force.

- Trepidation, harmony, stagnation, turmoil, stability, and bliss are the common phases of this journey. At any point in the program and at any phase, we can regroup and recommit to changing our destinies when we fall off the course.

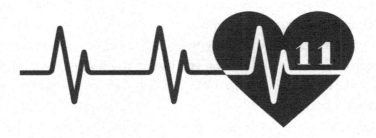

Kindle the Fire

As we discovered in chapter 9, agni is the basis of health, disease, and bliss. Imbalanced agni results in a system-wide neurohormonal imbalance that affects every cell of every organ system. As we have seen earlier, hormones are chemical substances that are released in response to the body's need for balance, or equilibrium. And equilibrium is a moment-to-moment assessment based on what we are thinking, feeling, and doing, which through the neurohormonal superhighways results in a cascade of effects. Hormones are released in response to our physical, emotional, and mental states, leading to subsequent chemical and neurological reactions that attempt to bring us back to equilibrium.

An imbalance in agni leads to several kinds of responses in the neurohormonal system. If the fire is fanned in an irregular fashion because of a vata imbalance, equilibrium is never steady. Balance and imbalance alternate rapidly, causing the nadis (energy channels) to dry up. Supporting and nourishing hormones become depleted, affecting the whole body and giving rise to a general sense of unrest, nonspecific aches and pains, and irregular bowel movements and sleep. If the fire takes over the system, it burns everything in its path, and the nadis (channels) begin to singe and shut down. Stress hormones become overactive and dominate over the supporting hormones, leading to chronic irritability, anger, heartburn and inability to look at situations in a calm manner. If the fire remains feeble, the neurohormonal system becomes underactive. The quality of the supporting hormones is tarnished by an underactive agni, leading to laziness, weight gain, improper digestion and loss of motivation. If unchecked, any of the imbalances lead to full-blown diseases and take us further and further away from bliss.[28]

Regardless of what your imbalance is, we always begin with balancing vata. This is because vata is always the first principle to go out of balance and is the easiest to correct. Recall that vata is the principle of movement. Life is defined by movement, as we can see down to the microscopic level. Constant movement is required for the functioning of prana, which determines the function of electrical impulses traveling down nerve cells, the release of hormones and chemicals from the cells, interaction of various chemicals within the cell, taking in of nutrients and oxygen and giving out of waste and carbon dioxide, the arising and subsiding of thoughts and emotions, the beating of the heart, and the constant change that defines our lives. In short, everything that we associate with life is constantly in motion and is facilitated by vata, the king dosha.

Most often, simply bringing vata back into balance resolves most or all health ailments. For this reason, my Bliss Rx for balancing agni leans heavily toward first bringing vata into balance. Once this is achieved, the specific issues of agni being overactive (due to pitta imbalance) or underactive (due to kapha imbalance) can be worked out much more easily.

Since vata is about dynamism, the prescription for returning it to balance is simple, which is to maintain regularity in our daily schedules.

The Need for Regularity

Notice how nature maintains a regular schedule. Plants and animals have very regimented routines from day to day and from season to season. They have an inherent sense of timing, whether it has to do with feeding, eliminating, flowering, maturing, or mating. When seasons change they

---

28 To determine your specific imbalance and heal it, take my Blissful Gut quiz:
    http://kavithamd.com/blissful-gut-quiz/

adjust their routines accordingly, shedding or hibernating according to their particular needs.

One of the advantages of being human is that we can choose to act and think independently. We are not compelled by nature's rhythms and can defy them to create our own cycles of feeding, eliminating, and mating. Although this is of great advantage when it comes to living our lives in our chosen ways and contributes to the evolution of the human race, our hormones that remain attuned to our rhythms take a beating. When we eat and sleep at irregular times, the body compensates for a while before its stores of prana are gradually depleted. Stress hormones begin to predominate, remaining on guard for when they may be called into action. You may choose to have a meal at midnight, when the digestive system is naturally inclined to rest, which then calls out to the neurohormonal system to bail it out. Irregular routines are like building a campfire where there are gusts of wind; agni becomes irregular, leading to the haphazard release of hormones.

Such a situation is easily managed by the system for a while, considering how intelligent it is. The stores of prana, tejas, and ojas we have built up earlier come to our aid and enable us to breeze through them. Chronic irregularities dip into the stores and as they become depleted, we start to notice their effects. Consider how well you managed in college by surviving on coffee and a few hours of sleep. If you continued that lifestyle over years, you notice that it doesn't work as well anymore. You may attribute it to aging but can't explain the aches and pains you have all over the body, your erratic bowel movements, sleep problems, and, if you are a woman, the symptoms of bloating, pain, and irritability before periods or the disabling symptoms of menopause.

Take the example of Judy, a fifty-five-year-old woman who came to see me for a second opinion about her long list of symptoms. She had seen two other cardiologists, who had performed extensive testing and dismissed her as having no "real" health issues. She had chronic shortness of breath, trouble sleeping at night, frequent hot flashes even though she had gone through menopause nearly eight years prior, and chronic constipation. She had been gaining weight steadily over the years, with nearly fifty pounds in the last two. She was in tears as she told me that she knew it was not heart disease but was frustrated that nobody had found an answer to why she felt so miserable.

She was taking several supplements, including some Ayurvedic ones, and felt that none of them were working. I reviewed her history and all the testing she had gone through, concluding that the previous cardiologists had been right: she had no signs of heart disease. However, she had all the signs of an imbalanced agni. She ate three meals one day and fasted the next. She went to bed at 9 p.m. on some days and at 2 a.m. on others. She was unmotivated and lacked energy. I asked her if she was willing to try my recommendations, and she eagerly agreed. I asked her to stop all the supplements and follow a regimented routine, along with dietary modifications as in the next chapter. Giving her printed instructions, I asked her to return in two months.

When Judy came back, she appeared more well-rested. She had lost a few pounds, was sleeping better, and her constipation had resolved. She stated that although her energy had improved, she was still quite fatigued. Her agni was improving. I reassured her that lifestyle changes take time, then made a few more recommendations and asked her to return in a few months. When she came back some months later, she stated that she had fallen "off course" due to her husband's health problems that landed him in the hospital. She was back to her irregular habits, but she stated that this time she could see the difference between how she felt when she followed the program versus when she didn't. Only in retrospect did she realize how much better she had felt when she followed a regular routine.

As her agni came into balance, she began to have the ability to see the root cause of her health problems—her chronic anxiety and stress. She told me how she had been chronically stressed and worried about everything from her own health to that of her family, imagined future outcomes, and past events that no longer had meaning. She told me that until she got into a regular routine, she didn't even realize her stress or what had caused it!

Judy's story is typical. Until agni is balanced, we are often oblivious to the stressful ways in which we think and live. Tamas shrouds our ability to see our own disabling patterns. I often tell my patients that a regular routine is like having the culture of mandatory uniforms in high school. Wearing the same thing to school every day eliminates the stress and distraction of finding the "right thing" to wear at an age when appearance is crucial. Similarly, doing things at the same time every day creates the perfect milieu for the body to stop the erratic flow of hormones and allow them to settle down into a predictable pattern. Once this happens, the whole system breathes a sigh of relief and can turn to other housekeeping items, such as figuring out the source of stress and eliminating it. If the system is always on guard to put out fires, it can't figure out where the fire is coming from!

The principle of maintaining regularity is based upon our internal clocks, which are remarkably accurate.

The Highly Accurate Internal Clock

If you've ever traveled across time zones, you've experienced the effects of jet lag on your body, including your energy level, digestion, sleep cycles, and a general feeling of disruption. You may also recall that it took several days to return to normal, depending upon how many time zones you crossed. Jet lag is one of the most obvious signs of our surprisingly accurate biological clocks, which are responsible for the balance between tissue building and breakdown that occur in cycles perfectly synchronized with light. We now know the workings of these clocks due to the highly active scientific field of chronobiology.

Remember the hypothalamus, the part of the brain that coordinates hormonal, immune, and autonomic nervous systems of the body? In this hard-working part of the brain there is a group of nerve cells called supra-chiasmatic nuclei (SCN), which is the master clock of the body. The SCN is entrained by several external cues known as zeitgebers (German: *zeit*= time, *geber*=keeper) to synchronize with the earth's twenty-four-hour cycle. The strongest zeitgeber is light, others being eating, sleeping, social interactions, seasons, and temperature. However, the SCN works even without the influence of zeitgebers. This means that your SCN nerve cells would continue to fire precisely and efficiently in approximately twenty-four-hour cycles for weeks, months, or years even if you stayed in complete darkness with no external cues!

Not only is the SCN an integral part of human physiology, it has evolved across various species including plants, fungi, and animals. Proteins known as cryptochromes are found in plants and in the eyes of humans and animals. These proteins are activated by light and send a signal to the SCN, which begins orchestrating the various neurohormonal pathways. For instance, the electrical impulse from light at dawn signals the SCN to "switch off" melatonin secretion from the pineal gland and "switch on" cortisol from the adrenals. Melatonin is the "sleepy" hormone that induces sleep, while cortisol gets the body ready for the day.

By isolating day and night within the body's systems, we can isolate the building (anabolic) and expending (catabolic) functions of the body, which is like separating the gas and brake pedals in a car. If we press both pedals at the same time, we wouldn't get too far. As we go about engaging with the world during the day and withdrawing from it at night, our two diametrically opposing forms of metabolism are kept separate by our internal clocks. Anabolic functions of tissue building and repair occur best at night, while catabolic functions of expending energy happen during the day.

These switches occur seamlessly from day to night by the rise and fall of the different hormones that are responsible for cell growth, heart rate and blood pressure changes, activation of the heart and vascular system, kidney and digestive functions, tissue metabolism, and release of cellular waste products. We now know that all body functions are subject to the circadian rhythm and considering the prevalence of the circadian rhythm in the plant and animal kingdom, we see that it is an evolutionary benefit—it gives us the opportunity to take advantage of the day and night for optimal functioning of our systems.

The Clock Mechanism

The SCN controls hormonal cycles and metabolic rhythms in two ways. Through its connection with the brain center that controls sleep and wakefulness, it determines the time you go to sleep, how long you sleep, and when you wake up. It also controls the secretion of nocturnal hormones such as prolactin and growth hormone that are anabolic in their actions. Independent of sleep, the SCN clock connects to the hormonal and autonomic nervous systems, which maintain functions like body temperature. This is how your body temperature rises and falls even when you are jet lagged and sleep deprived. If your body temperature depended entirely upon sleep, you wouldn't be able to travel!

The SCN isn't the only center in the body that maintains a twenty-four-hour clock in the body. All major organ systems including the liver, heart, kidneys, and skeletal muscles have clock mechanisms known as "oscillators." Upon detecting the first exposure to light, the SCN sends signals to these oscillators that then become synchronized to the circadian rhythm and to each other, maintaining functions such as hunger, wakefulness, respiration, and digestion. The SCN not only synchronizes our lifestyle, habits, hormonal, and autonomic systems to day-and-night cycles but also influences the tissue clocks. In turn, the tissue clocks drive cyclical gene expression of metabolism and physiology, detoxification and tissue building.

Recall that genes carry information for the body to encode all the proteins required for the functioning of the body. Clock cells have been found to act via two gene families known as period and cryptochrome. At the beginning of the day cycle, the clock cell nuclei begin the process of encoding these two genes where their RNAs begin to accumulate within the cell (recall that RNA is the intermediary between DNA and protein).[29] RNAs enable the creation of the proteins that rise slowly in the cell throughout the day. By the end of the day, the protein level peaks in

---

29 The Nobel Prize in Physiology or Medicine 2017 was awarded jointly to Jeffrey C. Hall, Michael Rosbash, and Michael W. Young for their discoveries of molecular mechanisms controlling the circadian rhythm: https://www.nobelprize.org/nobel_prizes/medicine/laureates/2017/

the cell, sending a signal for a fall in the RNA levels. This starts the night cycle. This loop is supported by the beginning and ending of activation of hundreds of other SCN genes that control several neuronal functions. A rare disorder of one of the SCN genes is known to cause a sleep disorder, and damage to the SCN can cause heart rhythm and other disorders.

Our bodies function at their best when all our organ systems follow circadian cycles in rhythm with each other and with the sun and the seasons. Knowing how our bodies follow the day-and-night cycles helps us understand the surge of certain diseases during specific times of the day or during particular seasons. For instance, the internal clock kicks up cardiovascular activity upon waking up, preparing us for the day. Heart attacks and strokes are more common early in the day, when the clock causes a rise in cortisol and other hormones that increase heart rate and blood pressure. Poor sleep hygiene (staying up late; consuming alcohol, caffeine, or large meals; using electronics and other stimulating media before bed) is known to have an impact on cellular metabolism and mental health, including insulin resistance, high blood pressure, high cholesterol, and a predisposition toward cardiovascular disease.

Shift Work

Shift work is common and required in many industries due to the need for twenty-four-hour coverage of duties. Many studies have shown the detrimental effects of shift work, raising important questions about the practice on workers' health. In one recent study, researchers used simulated laboratory conditions to mimic shift work in volunteers where their sleep-wake cycles were moved by twelve hours every three days (which is quite a common routine among shift workers), finding that this misalignment caused several alarming cardiovascular changes.[30] Even after they accounted for the participants' risk factors, a disruption in circadian rhythm led to increased blood pressure, decreased heart rate variability, and increased inflammatory markers in the blood. What is astounding

---

30 C. J. Morris, T. E. Purvis, K. Hu, and F. A. Scheer, "Circadian misalignment increases cardiovascular disease risk factors in humans," *Proc Natl Acad Sci USA* 113 (2016): E1402–11.

about this study is that these changes occurred over a very short period of time—the entire study took place over two eight-day intervals. Other studies have shown similar findings; as a result, shift work is considered a hidden risk factor for heart disease. Jerry was a striking example of the effects of shift working on the heart.

He had been working night shifts as a security guard for twenty years when he came to see me for high blood pressure. Even after two decades of the "upside down" routine, as he called it, his body-mind wasn't accustomed to it. He was tired all the time, and his blood pressure was creeping up over the years. We had a long discussion about his routine. Realizing that it was contributing to his deteriorating health, Jerry said he would think about finding another job. I gave him a prescription for a blood pressure–lowering medicine. A year later he found another job with regular working hours, and almost overnight his outlook toward life changed. Gradually his blood pressure went down, and eventually I took him off his medicine. He is a changed man with abundant energy and positivity, traits that were uncovered when his circadian rhythm normalized.

Shift workers have been shown to have a higher risk for other serious concerns, such as cancer, but these risks are not entirely related to lack of sleep. Even if you get enough sleep, the misalignment with your internal clock is enough to cause serious health concerns. Although there are some medications to help with excessive sleepiness among shift workers, there are no effective therapies at this time to lower the risk for health problems.

While modern medicine presents us with exciting possibilities for understanding disease and therapy, the circadian rhythm should give us reason to pause and wonder—what is the driving force for the activation of the genes? What diurnal and seasonal forces enable the efficient functioning of the body-mind? We tend to come up short when we ask these fundamental questions. However, if we turn to Ayurveda, we are presented with a cohesive theory that answers these questions in a holistic fashion. Once again, it comes down to the three doshas.

Driving Forces of the Internal Clock

Recall that the doshas are the hidden puppeteers of the body-mind, arising from the five elements and combining in specific ways (chapter 8). Now let's take a broader look at the doshas and how they determine our internal clocks.

Everything in nature is cyclical, as we readily see in the changing of seasons, day and night patterns, and the growth and decay of the human body. These cycles are maintained and propelled by the three doshas. It helps to think of their properties to understand how they function throughout our lives and in nature.

Vata is a combination of air and space. If you think of the properties of air and space, what vata does will become apparent. Air is light and is characterized by movement and lightness. Thus, it is quick, dry, and cold. Like space, vata is subtle. It predominates in the fall and early winter when the weather is cool and dry. Pitta is a combination of fire and water, giving it the properties of heat, oiliness, and quickness. It is the predominant dosha in the summer months. Kapha, which is the combination of water and earth, is heavy, unctuous, and cold. It predominates in late winter and spring.

Our life cycles are also subject to the doshas. Kapha is the dosha of childhood, marked by growth, grounding, and nourishment. Adulthood is characterized by pitta, where we are driven by the "fire in the belly" to live a life of purpose and to pay bills, enjoy pleasures of the senses, and contribute to society. Vata is the dosha of old age, characterized by dryness of joints and tissues, onset of various illnesses, and general deterioration.

Daily dosha cycles mimic those of our life cycles, where kapha predominates at the beginning of the day, pitta at midday, and vata at the end of the day, repeating every twelve hours:

Vata: 2–6 a.m. and 2–6 p.m.

Pitta: 10 a.m.–2 p.m. and 10 p.m.–2 a.m.

Kapha: 6–10 a.m. and 6–10 p.m.

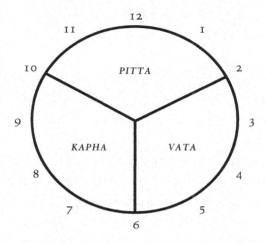

Figure 5: The "Dosha Clock." This represents times of the day when each dosha is most active.

Note that these are approximate times and that all three doshas are always present; it is just that one of them predominates over the other two around these particular times. Once again, let's take a look at the properties of the doshas, which will help us understand how they influence our internal clocks. Remember that vata is the principle of movement—it moves impulses required for all aspects of the circadian rhythm, carrying information of light or dark to the internal clocks, regulating the release of the various hormones in accordance with daily, seasonal, and life cycles. The movement of vata drives the functions of pitta and kapha, ordering the mind's activity with time, determining aging in relation to time, pushing us to be motivated at certain times and to wind down at others, and, importantly, maintaining homeostasis.

Vata drives the release or withdrawal of key hormones that initiate the cycles of metabolism and tissue repair. Production of serotonin, adrenaline (or epinephrine), and glucocorticoids begin in the morning vata time. Serotonin brings us back to the waking state after a night's rest while adrenaline and glucocorticoids begin to wake up the brain and other organs. Glucocorticoids initiate the release of glucose stored in the liver cells for energy and metabolic processes. Metabolism begins to slow down by the end of the evening vata time as the body begins to prepare for rest.

Kapha regulates structure, water balance, and the growth and strength of organs, tissues, cells, and the mind. Spurred into action by vata, kapha responds to the hormones produced in the morning—for instance, the breakdown of glucose by glucocorticoids initiates the delicate dance between the pancreas and the liver that produce insulin and glucagon to maintain balance. Insulin regulates not only glucose metabolism but also cell growth. Kapha times are characterized by a reconstituting of metabolic functions into equilibrium, where the breaking down and building up of structures are balanced. At kapha-predominant times there is an increased predilection for rebuilding body structures and sustained energy for prolonged activity.[31]

Pitta regulates transformation through digestion and metabolism. Urged by vata, pitta begins its actions on the released hormones with a steady increase in body temperature and metabolism in the form of the countless cellular reactions throughout the organs that peak by midday. Hunger is initiated by the action of pitta on the liver and digestive organs that are primed to release their enzymes with meal intake. During its predominance from 10 p.m. to 2 a.m., pitta regulates the scavenging of free radicals (byproducts of cellular metabolism) by the actions of melatonin, the pineal gland hormone that induces the night cycle. While pitta during its morning cycle regulates catabolic actions for release and expenditure of energy, it governs anabolic functions at night, including tissue repair.

Using Our Clocks to Balance Agni

The two most important things we can do to balance agni are to maintain regular sleep and meal times. Let's look at the mechanisms by which each of these work.

---

31 A. Hankey, "A test of the systems analysis underlying the scientific theory of Ayurveda's Tridosha," *J Altern Complement Med* 11 (2005): 385–90.

Maintain Regular Sleep Times

We have seen the various effects of the sleep-wake cycle upon our internal clocks. Looking at sleep and wake times through the lens of the doshas might help us understand this recommendation further.

Wake up no later than 6 a.m. and go to bed no later than 10 p.m. Now that you've seen the daily cycles of the doshas, this recommendation will make more sense. Vata, as we saw earlier, predominates until 6 a.m. Here's the thing about vata: since it is made of up space and air, its subtle actions are more evident on the mind than in the body. It governs creativity, enthusiasm, and cognitive abilities, which peak during vata times. Waking up when vata predominates fosters these abilities; studying or meditating during this period is much more effective than during other times. Since vata also governs elimination, waking up before 6 a.m. regulates your bowels.

Recall that kapha is the combination of water and earth; its essential qualities are heaviness, slowness, and dullness. This is why we feel groggy or fog-headed when we wake up during the morning kapha time. We lose the advantages that vata offers with waking up late, including mental clarity and elimination.

On the other hand, kapha is very conducive to sleep at night because of the very qualities that make it unfavorable for waking up late in the morning. Recall that pitta revs up our metabolism and becomes active at 10 p.m., which is why sleep problems are common with what is known as "night vigil," or staying up too late. Going to sleep in the kapha time ensures better rest and deeper sleep.

A common question that arises from this prescription is this—what does this mean for those of us who are not "morning types"? While we may consider ourselves to be morning or evening types, recent research is demonstrating the wisdom of going to bed early and waking up early. For instance, one study among adolescents showed that later bedtimes and waking times are associated with obesity and lower physical fitness regardless of other factors such as how much sleep they got.[32] "Evening-ness" also affects overall quality of life and physical and mental health, as well as performance at school and at work.[33]

Maintain Regular Mealtimes

Eating your meals at the same time is like feeding the campfire with a steady supply of firewood when a steady fire is the desired result. Main-taining a reasonable gap between meals is like allowing the fire to con-sume a log before burdening it with another. When we eat on time, the neurohormonal system of the gut is regularized so the system becomes used to secreting the needed juices and enzymes at the same intervals. When we eat about the same quantity of food, we enable the system to work without over- or under-producing the required juices. Overproduc-tion of gastric acid leads to heartburn, when the agni is out of control and there is not enough good-quality fuel for the campfire. Underproduction of digestive juices leads to indigestion and, eventually, disease.

Here are some general considerations:

- Eat (light) breakfast between 7 and 8 a.m.
- Eat (heavy) lunch between 10 a.m. and 2 p.m.
- Eat (light) dinner no later than 6:30 p.m.

Let's revisit the doshas and why these recommendations might make sense. Breakfast rolls around in the kapha time. Recall that although our catabolic hormones are rising, kapha's heavy qualities predominate over the body-mind and, consequently, over agni. Most of us may not be par-ticularly hungry during this time, thanks to the actions of kapha on the digestive system. However, despite a lack of appetite, the body requires nourishment and substrate for the actions of the catabolic hormones (and agni) that are beginning to rise. A light breakfast fulfills this need and keeps our energy levels up while pacifying agni.

---

32 T. S. Olds, C. A. Maher, and L. Matricciani, "Sleep duration or bedtime? Exploring the relationship between sleep habits and weight status and activity patterns," *Sleep* 34 (2011): 1299–307.

33 F. Fabbian, B. Zucchi, A. De Giorgi, et al., "Chronotype, gender and general health," *Chronobiol Int* 33 (2016): 863–82.

Pitta kicks in around 10 a.m. and drives up our metabolism. Juices and enzymes in the digestive tract are at their peak in the daytime pitta period, coinciding with our largest appetite and hunger. Agni burns bright in the pitta time since they both are defined by heat. The largest meal of the day must thus be eaten at midday, when our digestive capacities are at their optimal levels.

Our evening meals tend to coincide with kapha and vata times, when the hormonal systems begin to turn metabolism from catabolic to anabolic processes. For instance, the same pitta that drives hunger and digestion at midday drives detoxification while the body is at rest at night. Since the body is winding down and preparing for rest during the evening kapha time when it is dinner time for most of us, eating a heavy meal results in agni imbalance and production of ama. Studies have shown that eating large meals in the evening has deleterious effects on insulin metabolism, which reverses when the eating cycle is changed to take in the majority of the day's calories during daytime.[34]

This is one recommendation that many of my patients find difficult, particularly when they are accustomed to eating their heaviest meals in the evening. However, the significance of this recommendation cannot be overstated when we consider the implications of consuming large meals at the end of the day. The longer the duration of nighttime fasting, the lower is the propensity for inflammation and insulin resistance. In one study, reducing evening caloric intake and eating early to increase nighttime fasting was associated with lower levels of C-reactive protein, the marker associated with inflammation, atherosclerosis, heart disease, and cancers.[35]

---

34 D. Jakubowicz, M. Barnea, J. Wainstein, and O. Froy, "High caloric intake at breakfast vs. dinner differentially influences weight loss of overweight and obese women," *Obesity (Silver Spring)* 21 (2013): 2504–12.

35 C. R. Marinac, D. D. Sears, L. Natarajan, L. C. Gallo, C. I. Breen, and R. E. Patterson, "Frequency and circadian timing of eating may influence biomarkers of inflammation and insulin resistance associated with breast cancer risk," *PLoS One* 10 (2015): e0136240.

Working with Your Body-Mind Rhythm

While regularizing eating and sleeping times is the most important thing
we can do to bring agni back to balance, we can use the knowledge of
the doshas to our advantage in regulating the following elements of our
lifestyles as well:

Exercise

The best time to exercise is 6–10 a.m., when physical activity counters
the natural presence of kapha's heaviness and slowness in the context of
the rising levels of catabolic processes. On the other hand, heavy exercise
in the evening kapha period, when the body is winding down with the
onset of anabolic processes, causes agni imbalance over the long term.
Routinely exercising during the highly catabolic pitta period also causes
an agni imbalance, with a tendency toward inflammatory conditions, irritability, anger, stress, restlessness, and so on.

Regulating Agni During Menstruation

The cyclic process of menstruation is driven by the three doshas that
predominate at various times during the cycle. The first two weeks after
menses are governed by kapha, when the uterine lining begins to rebuild
itself. Ovulation marks the beginning of the pitta period, when the lining
becomes engorged with blood in preparation for the fertilized egg. If conception does not occur, vata sets menses in motion. Menstruation has the
immense advantage of periodically cleansing the body of ama. The rise in
heart disease with the onset of menopause also coincides with the loss of
ama cleansing and its subsequent accumulation. In women, imbalanced
agni presents itself as an imbalance in menstruation, resulting in almost
all disorders of the body-mind. And the most important remedy for the
imbalance is to regulate the circadian rhythm beginning at menarche; see
the resources section for some excellent books on a holistic approach to
women's health.

During menstruation, in addition to maintaining regular timings, we
can pay special attention to lifestyle choices to aid vata's work of cleansing. Strenuous activity and exercise results in an increase in heart rate,

respiration, and blood flow to the skeletal muscles (among many other things), all of which are mediated by vata moving in specific directions. During menstruation, vata naturally flows in a downward fashion (just as it does during bowel movements, urination, and childbirth). Strenuous exercise while menstruating results in a vata "steal" due to conflicting flows. Over time, this results in an imbalanced agni. Instead, plenty of rest helps with optimal vata functioning and a balanced menstrual cycle, which is defined as having no discomfort or premenstrual symptoms, moderate flow of bright red blood that doesn't stain clothing, and lack of mood swings. A balanced agni also manifests as a trouble-free menopause with no hot flashes, mood swings, or irregularities.

From a holistic perspective, this makes total sense since menstruation and menopause are governed by sex hormones as we explored in chapter 6, which in turn respond adversely to external or internal stress.

Take One Step at a Time

If you're a night owl or have a tendency to fast all day and gorge at night, the above recommendations may be difficult to implement. If you try to do it all at once, it may even throw your system out of balance temporarily, so I suggest taking it slowly.

Begin to make small changes in your sleep/wake times, perhaps by 15–30 minutes every few days. For instance, if you are accustomed to a bedtime of midnight and waking up at 7:30 a.m., begin by going to bed at 11:45 p.m. and waking up at 7:15 a.m. After a few days, sleep at 11:30 p.m. and wake up at 7 a.m. Continue to change your schedule gradually until you get to the recommended times.

Similarly, if you're used to skipping lunch and having a heavy dinner, start by eating a small lunch and a slightly lighter meal at night. Wait for several days for your system to get used to this schedule before making further changes. In the next chapter we will see what to eat for health and bliss.

Summary

- Imbalanced agni results in a system-wide neurohormonal imbalance that affects the functioning of all body-mind functions.

- Regardless of the type of agni imbalance, balancing vata is of crucial importance. Most often, simply bringing vata back into balance resolves most or all health ailments and is based on the circadian rhythm.

- The circadian rhythm of the body-mind is regulated by a master clock in the hypothalamus and molecular clocks in the cells of various organs that switch their functions seamlessly from day to night by the rise and fall of the different hormones.

- Our body-minds function at their optimal level when we are in sync with cycles of day and night and the seasons.

- Chronically being out of sync with these cycles (such as in shift work) results in a depletion of prana, tejas, and ojas, the fine essences of cellular metabolism, resulting in disease.

- Our life cycles, seasons, and diurnal rhythms are regulated by the three doshas, which are the basis of the Bliss Rx for sleeping and eating schedules.

- Waking up before 6 a.m. and going to bed by 10 p.m. optimizes the workings of the body-mind.

- Eating the largest meal of the day at midday and a light, early dinner helps balance agni and decrease inflammation and risks for various chronic illnesses.

- The best time to exercise is 6–10 a.m., when physical activity counters the natural presence of heaviness and slowness of kapha in the context of the rising levels of catabolic processes.

- Strenuous exercise while menstruating interferes with the normal flow of vata and results in agni imbalance.
- Making schedule changes gradually is better for long-term adherence.

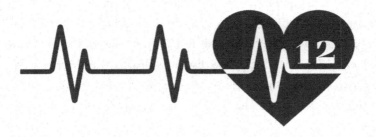

Eat for Bliss

What you will learn in this chapter might surprise you. We have seen earlier that magic bullets don't exist, particularly when it comes to diet and lifestyle choices. Moreover, what works for one person will not work for another since "diet" is more about what we are able to digest than what we can eat, and what we are able to digest depends entirely on the state of our agni. Let me illustrate this point by telling you the story of two patients, Bill and Peter.

I first met Bill after he had a minor heart attack during knee surgery at age fifty-four. Prior to the heart attack, he had no symptoms or signs of heart disease except for high cholesterol. However, the stress of the surgery and this new diagnosis threw him over the edge and his blood pressure shot up, remaining consistently high over weeks and months. When I met him in the office, he was determined to do whatever he could to "fight" his heart disease and insisted that I counsel him about the best possible diet for him. I recommended a low-fat plant-based diet considering its cholesterol-lowering and anti-inflammatory benefits, giving him extensive resources and literature to read up on and sending him to a nutritionist for in-depth counseling.

When I saw him in follow-up six months later, I could barely recognize him. He had lost twenty-five pounds without trying, and his LDL cholesterol had dipped so low that I lowered his statin dose. His wife was very concerned about his weight loss and wondered if he would get "too thin." I reassured them both that his body would find equilibrium and that there was no need to worry. I was so pleased with his progress that I was surprised when he made an unscheduled appointment two months later. He was still on the diet and had no symptoms of heart disease, but he and his wife were deeply unhappy that he had given up so much of their beloved foods such as meat and desserts. He confessed that he was very conflicted; on one hand he saw how well the diet had worked, and on the other he felt that his social and family lives were deteriorating because of it. When I suggested that he ease up on the diet and enjoy his favorite foods once in a while, he shook his head in fear. He did not want another heart attack at any cost.

Bill made another unscheduled appointment three months later. His numbers were still looking good and he was still asymptomatic, but he was more miserable this time. His wife was visibly upset and admitted that his diet had become a nidus for stress in their marriage. This time, I sat down with both of them and firmly asked Bill to quit the diet. The benefits of the diet were being overwhelmed by the stress of the social and family situation it caused. I told him that it was simply not worth it and that it would be much better for his heart if he were happy and content while taking medications than being chronically stressed on no medications. This time he seemed relieved, like he was being freed from prison. On subsequent visits, Bill seemed like a changed man. Although he regained some body weight and was back on a higher dose of statins, his more cheerful outlook indicated a happier life.

Now take the example of Peter, whom I met when he accompanied his wife, Emma, on her visit to my office. She had no evidence of heart disease herself but had a very strong history of it in her family. At forty-eight she was nearing menopause and wanted to know what she could do to lower her risk for heart disease. I went over my lifestyle recommendations with her and talked to her about a plant-based diet. Peter, who had been listening intently, began to ask me questions about the diet. At fifty years of age he had already had several stents and open-heart surgery for coronary artery disease. He was a patient of one of my partners and had seen several other doctors for lifestyle and diet recommendations. He said he had never heard about the benefits of a plant-based diet and wanted to know more. As with Bill, I gave Peter and Emma several resources on the topic.

Several months later I was waiting in line at the hospital coffee shop when a man strode up to me and gave me a big hug. It was Peter, and I could barely recognize him. He had lost nearly thirty pounds on the plant-based diet and said that everyone in his family, including his young grandchildren, had adopted it. He was thriving on the diet, with boundless energy, better sleep, and an improved state of mind. A year later he saw his doctor in a routine follow-up, and his blood pressure and cholesterol were so low that he was taken off all medicines except for aspirin.

Bill and Peter (and countless other patients) have taught me that what is nectar for one is poison for another. I no longer recommend the same diet for everyone and instead look at what eating habits would bring out the best in each patient's body-mind. More importantly, I recommend incorporating the suggestions laid out in this chapter that balance agni and facilitate remembrance of our true blissful nature by regulating our neurohormonal pathways.

Dietary Practices of the Bliss Model

The principles of balancing agni with diet are to both regulate neurohormonal pathways and optimize the power of digestive juices. Pathways of any kind depend on vata, the principle of movement, while digestive juices—with their ability to transform food into body constituents—invoke the function of pitta. As with regulating our daily rhythms, balancing vata takes precedence. Balancing vata enables the free flow of prana through the countless channels of the subtle body. A balanced metabolism (pitta) ensures radiance (tejas) and that the prana channels don't shrivel up from lack of its heat or burn from too much of it. Unobstructed flow of prana enables complete digestion and metabolism with no ama residue and the production of ojas, the substance of bliss. While some of these recommendations may seem familiar, others may sound completely unconventional.

Regulate Neurohormonal Pathways

The following recommendations consider the principles of balancing the free flow of vata that are critical for electrical and chemical impulses to travel from cell to cell and from organ to organ. When vata becomes stagnant or obstructed, pathways become erratic and dysfunctional, resulting in incomplete digestion of food, sensory information, thoughts, memories, and emotions. This body-mind imbalance is not conducive to knowing our true blissful self. Imbalance keeps us fixated on the body-mind as the source of our pain and joy, which as we have seen is the basic misunderstanding that leads to suffering. When we pay attention to what we eat and how we eat, these pathways reclaim their smooth flow.

The general principles of regulating neurohormonal pathways through diet are to avoid difficult to digest foods, favor simple foods that nourish the body-mind, and follow proper eating etiquette that respects the workings of the pathways. Although it seems like hard work initially, a peculiar thing begins to happen when the body-mind pathways reinvigorate—we will know what to eat simply by listening to the body, and we will have developed the ability to differentiate between habits and need, craving and nourishment.

A note about scientific studies regarding diet: if you were to dig through PubMed (a database of published studies), you will find conflicting studies regarding particular foods. Take coffee, for instance, which has been found to be proinflammatory and harmful as a risk factor in chronic illnesses in some studies and beneficial in others as an anti-inflammatory agent. How come? Remember the observer bias we examined in chapter 2, where the fundamental problem in studying a phenomenon is that it changes its behavior simply because it is being observed? Besides, in the example of coffee, it may be beneficial for you and harmful for me because of our unique neurohormonal wiring that is based on our biology and how we think, feel, act, and live.

Many of the recommendations here may be dismissed by nutritionists, doctors, and healthcare professionals as being unscientific. I had dismissed them as well until I put them to the test myself. Most importantly, scientific studies are performed in the default model based on the premise that the body-mind is who we are; I know this all too well because scientific research is part of my job.

The recommendations below are based on the bliss model and on the premise that establishing balance in the body-mind makes it conducive for us to discover our true nature. We may (or may not) find studies to support some of these recommendations. Perhaps we are lagging a bit and the studies will eventually be performed, just as depression and shift work were described thousands of years ago to be harmful but are only recently being recognized in modern medicine as risk factors for chronic illness. My suggestion would be to try the recommendations in this chapter yourself. Give it a fair chance by following them for a few months, and draw your own conclusions.

Here are the most important dietary recommendations to get you established on your path to bliss:

- Avoid inflammatory substances such as refined sugars (cakes, cookies, pastries, and other products), yeasted breads and baked goods, trans fats and red meats. Refined starches, sugar, saturated fats, excess dairy, red and processed meats have been shown to promote inflammation.[36]

- Favor freshly prepared and fully cooked meals with simple ingredients. Recall that everything in creation pulsates with prana, the blissful life force. Stale, frozen, processed, and reheated foods lose prana rapidly along

---

36 D. Giugliano, A. Ceriello, and K. Esposito, "The effects of diet on inflammation: emphasis on the metabolic syndrome," *J Am Coll Cardiol* 48 (2006): 677–85.

with their nutritional value. This is why fresh foods taste better! Cooking with simple spices makes food palatable as well as more digestible.

- Avoid excess salt. Not only does excess salt cause an imbalance in the body's electrolytes and water balance, leading to neurohormonal imbalance (and can lead to difficulty controlling high blood pressure and heart failure), but it causes excessive strain on the subtle body and cause obstructions in the flow of prana, tejas, and ojas. Use unprocessed salt (such as Himalayan salt) that contains all the trace minerals and is not exposed to chemicals. Avoid adding salt to food that is already cooked. Adding it during cooking has the advantage of allowing the heat to carry the salt into the food, and therefore we require less of it.

- Avoid drinking water an hour before and an hour after meals. In order to balance agni, we need to optimize the workings of our digestive juices, which become diluted if consumed with meals. If needed, take sips of warm or room-temperature water. In general, drink only when thirsty; allow the body to tell you when to eat or drink.

- Avoid cold and raw foods and drinks. This is a recommendation that many Americans might have difficulty with because our culture here is to routinely add ice to beverages. Remember that these recommendations are to first and foremost balance vata. The general principle of food and lifestyle issues is that like increases like—vata is cold and dry and will become aggravated with anything that is similar. Cold drinks, particularly with meals and during cool months, can rapidly get the body-mind out of balance due to an imbalanced agni. Cold and raw foods like salads and cereals have the same effect. Choose warm and moist foods that counter the effects of vata. A small salad for lunch on occasion will do no harm if dressed in a healthy oil. Avoid salads at dinner. Sautéing or steaming vegetables makes them more digestible without aggravating vata. Often this simple change is enough to result in significant results, as Anna discovered. She is a fifty-five-year old executive who participated in the Heal Your Heart program. She had been trying to lose weight for years, sticking to salads for lunch every day. When she heard about the principle of agni imbalance, she immediately switched from cold salads to warm soups for lunch and sipped warm water or Bliss tea (recipe ahead) throughout the day. Within six months she had lost nearly fifteen pounds with no other change in her lifestyle.

- Avoid potatoes, cabbage, cauliflower, and brussel sprouts. All foods have inherent doshas in addition to their nutritional value. Although cruciferous vegetables have thyroid gland–enhancing nutritional content, they are high in vata.

- Minimize caffeine; better still, cut it out entirely. Although caffeine is shown to be of some benefit in certain medical conditions, it can lead to an overactive agni and the mental state of rajas, with restlessness, irritability, impatience, anger, sleep disturbance, and a disruption of our internal clocks. Coffee increases cortisol secretion that in turn leads to increased levels of insulin, which is inflammatory. It also dumbs down the cells' ability to process sugar by not responding to insulin, which can lead to metabolic syndrome of obesity, increased blood sugar, high blood pressure and triglycerides and decreased good cholesterol. Besides, if you have become habituated to coffee, you will realize how addictive it is. When I gave up my morning cup, I felt like a drug addict going through withdrawal, which was an accurate description! Relying on external substances for our happiness is the default model and is not conducive to the discovery of bliss.

- Always sit down to eat. Avoid watching TV, arguing, or excitation during meals. We have seen what happens in stress, where the body-mind prepares to deal with it. Blood flow is directed toward the arms and legs to take action, and flow to the digestive tract decreases. The body has better things to do in times of stress than digest food. The result of this sympathetic activation is indigestion. Sitting down relaxes us and keeps us focused on the task of eating. Pleasant conversation or, better yet, silent savoring of every bite aids digestion and calms agni.

- In Ayurveda we are asked to avoid combining certain foods because of their energetic properties that throw agni out of balance. Consume fruit and milk on their own and not with meals since their properties conflict with those of other foods.

- Use spices. Judicious use of spices not only makes food palatable but also helps with digestion. See ahead for a healing spice mix recipe that you can use in any dish.

Bliss-Promoting Recipes

Bliss Tea

Instead of iced water, try sipping this tea throughout the day. Take a sip or two every half hour or so. If you are still thirsty, drink small amounts of water at room temperature. Avoid drinking water before and after meals (see page 170). Stop sipping the tea at sunset or before dinner, whichever comes first.

Bring a quart of water to boil. Add a half teaspoon each of cumin, coriander, and fennel seeds, and let them steep for a few minutes. Strain into a thermos.

Agni Kindler

If you have an underactive agni, this recipe is for you. Avoid it if your agni is overactive and you have heartburn or diarrhea.

Grate 1 inch of fresh ginger. Mix with a teaspoon of lemon juice and a pinch of salt. Store in refrigerator. Chew on half a teaspoon of the mixture 10–30 minutes before lunch and dinner.

Ama Banisher

If you have signs of ama (constipation with sticky stools, bad breath, a thick coating on the tongue, a feeling of being bloated or blocked), this recipe is for you. Drink this mix first thing in the morning on an empty stomach.

To a cup of lukewarm (not hot) water, add a teaspoon of raw, unheated honey and a teaspoon of lemon juice. Mix well.

Honey, when raw and unheated, is medicine and promotes clarity and lightness. When heated, the enzymes, amino acids, and other beneficial substances in it are degraded. Not only is its medicinal property lost, but consuming heated or processed honey promotes further ama and stagnation—hence the suggestion to never heat honey. Here is an example of the same substance being medicine or poison depending on how you use it!

Bliss Spice Mix

Spices are generally underrated for their ability to heal and promote wellness. When used in the right combinations, spices not only add flavor to food but begin to affect our body-minds by bringing agni back to balance.

This versatile spice mix can be used in anything—soups, khichadi and dal (see ahead), oatmeal or other warm breakfast cereals, casseroles, and even sprinkled on cut fruit or vegetables.

Ingredients

> 5 teaspoons cumin
>
> 3 teaspoons coriander
>
> 5 teaspoons fennel
>
> 1 teaspoon black pepper
>
> ½ teaspoon fenugreek
>
> 1 teaspoon powdered ginger
>
> 1 teaspoon turmeric

Method

Grind to a powder in a coffee grinder and store in an airtight container. Alternatively, place the whole spices in a ceramic spice grinder and grind as much as you need directly into the dish while cooking. Add the ginger and turmeric powders separately. I love to use a mortar and pestle and freshly grind my spices while cooking. When short on time, I use the spice grinder.

Khichadi

If there is one recipe I'd recommend, it would be this. Khichadi has the consistency of a stew and is versatile because of the many variations in the ingredients. It is deeply satisfying and comforting, the combination of moong dal,[37] grains, and spices being sattvic and balancing. It is a staple lunch recipe in our home, where I prepare it fresh in the morning and

---

37 Moong dal is also called split green gram and is easily available in Asian grocery stores and in health food stores such as Whole Foods.

pack it in a thermos. It is a fantastic dish for cleansing, and I often eat only khichadi during times of intense spiritual practices, when I return home after travel, or when I feel overworked. This makes 2–3 generous lunch-sized servings.

Ingredients

　　1 cup basmati rice

　　1 cup moong dal

　　1 stick celery (optional)

　　1 inch fresh ginger

　　1–2 cups finely chopped vegetables of choice (such as
　　　　spinach or other greens, squash, green beans, sweet
　　　　potato, carrots)

　　1 teaspoon extra virgin olive oil

　　1–2 teaspoons bliss spice mix (adjust to taste)

　　1 teaspoon turmeric (if not part of the spice mix)

　　Salt to taste

Method

This dish is easier to prepare in a pressure cooker. If you don't have one, use a heavy-bottomed pan. Wash the rice and moong dal together several times under cold water and keep aside. Heat the oil in the pan and add the celery and ginger. When soft, add the spice mix and sauté for a minute. If using a spice grinder, add in the turmeric and the washed rice and dal mixture. Sauté for another minute. Add salt and three cups of water. Mix well (make sure to scrape the bottom) and bring to a boil. Turn the heat down and let it simmer until the mixture is mushy.[38] If

---

38　If using a stove-top pressure cooker, close the lid and let the pressure build up on high heat, then cook for 5 minutes on low heat. Take the cooker off the heat and let the pressure subside fully before opening. If using an electric cooker, close the lid and set the timer for 5 minutes, waiting for pressure to be released fully before opening it. Cooking times may vary depending upon the brand; you may have to experiment to figure out the best setting. I also use a slow cooker for this recipe on occasion. Once you've sautéed the mixture and added salt and water, transfer to a slow cooker and set it on high. Again, you may have to experiment to figure out the best settings for the consistency you like.

using vegetables like carrots or beans, add them in when the mixture is half done. If using greens, fold them in after the khichadi is cooked.

The khichadi will thicken when cooled. Add more water if desired to get a stew-like consistency. It is best eaten fresh and warm.

Variations

- Replace rice with other grains such as quinoa, millet, barley, cracked wheat, or brown rice
- Replace moong dal with red lentils or whole green gram (also available in Asian or health food stores)
- Vary the vegetables
- Try different spices, including fresh herbs such as cilantro, basil, rosemary, or thyme

Spiced Cream of Wheat

This dish, a staple in the part of the world where I grew up, is called upma. It is a standard breakfast fare, but I like it for brunch or lunch with a lot of vegetables. Like khichadi, it is versatile and easy to prepare.

Ingredients

1 cup Cream of Wheat (the coarser variety)

1 small onion, finely chopped

1 inch ginger, finely minced

1 teaspoon cumin seeds

1 teaspoon coriander seeds

1 cup vegetables of choice (peas, carrots, beans, shelled edamame, zucchini, etc.), finely chopped

2 teaspoons extra virgin olive oil

Black peppercorns to taste

Salt to taste

Juice of 1 lemon

Method

In a heavy bottomed pan, heat 1 teaspoon of the oil and pour in the Cream of Wheat. Sauté until it turns light brown and aromatic. Take it off the heat and pour into a lipped bowl or measuring cup. Heat the other teaspoon of oil and add the cumin, coriander, and peppercorns (cover with lid as the cumin tends to sputter). Add the onion and ginger and cook until soft, then add vegetables. Sauté for 2–3 minutes. Add 3 cups of water and the salt, and bring to a boil. Turn the heat down and very slowly pour in the Cream of Wheat while stirring continuously. Cover with lid and turn off the heat after a minute. Allow to cook in its own heat for a few minutes. Stir in the lemon juice and serve hot.

Optional: Add chopped herbs or shredded fresh coconut prior to
   serving.

Blissful Dal

This is another staple in my home because of its versatility and bliss-promoting properties. It can be had as a soup or made into a heavier meal when served over rice or other grains and with a side of vegetables. Full of high-quality protein, moong dal is easily digestible and very tasty.

Ingredients

   1 cup moong dal

   1 small onion, finely chopped

   1 inch ginger, finely minced

   2 garlic cloves, finely minced

   1 teaspoon extra virgin olive oil

   1–2 teaspoons bliss spice mix (adjust to taste)

   1 teaspoon turmeric (if not part of the spice mix)

   Salt to taste

   Juice of 1 lemon

Method

Wash the dal several times in cold water. Place in a heavy-bottomed pan with 4 cups of water. Bring to a boil and turn the heat down. Cook on low heat until dal is mushy (about 20–30 minutes). In a heavy-bottomed pan heat 1 teaspoon of the oil. Add the onion, ginger, and garlic and cook until soft, then add cooked dal, salt, turmeric (if not part of the spice mix), and spice mix. Add more water if needed. Allow to simmer for a few minutes. Stir in the lemon juice and serve hot over rice, quinoa, cracked wheat, or other grains.

Variations:

- Replace moong dal with red lentils
- Add steamed vegetables or fresh greens once dal is cooked
- Instead of the spice mix, add fresh or dried hot peppers to taste

Bliss Balls

Funny name notwithstanding, this is a super healthy dessert or midafternoon snack. Full of antioxidants and protein, it is so easy to prepare that you might end up making it often!

Ingredients

1½ cups pitted dates

1 cup mixed nuts such as almonds, cashews, and walnuts; avoid peanuts

½ cup coconut powder

Method

In a food processor, add the dates and nuts, then pulse until fine. Add a few drops of extra virgin olive oil if desired.

Take a handful of the mixture and roll by hand into tightly packed balls. Roll the balls in coconut powder.

Incorporating Bliss in Your Own Recipes

As you become more adept at following the guidelines of the program, have fun with your own creations within the context of your own culture and upbringing. Is there another way to cook Southern greens, for instance? Can you think of a different way to prepare simple foods like pasta, vegetables, or casseroles? Incorporate the spice mix and other spices liberally to change the textures and flavors of your own foods.

Remember to minimize the foods that cause havoc in our neurohormonal pathways and liberalize foods that are grounding and nurturing. In the resources section I've listed several cookbooks that employ such principles.

Sample Meal Plan

Breakfast

- Oatmeal, Cream of Wheat, or other hot cereal with bliss spice mix and a pinch of salt or with raisins and nuts
- Chopped sweet apple or pear cooked in water with 2 whole cloves or a stick of cinnamon, with or without raisins
- Cup of almond milk with ground cardamom and raw sugar to taste

Although spiced cereal sounds strange, it is a delicious alternative for those of us who don't like sweet tastes first thing in the morning.

Instead of oatmeal or Cream of Wheat, try this: put two tablespoons of cooked rice in a pot with a cup of water and bring it to a boil, then turn down the heat and cook for about 10 minutes. Mash with the back of a spoon and add either spice mix and salt or raisins and nuts.

For an extra nutritional boost, add a tablespoon of flaxseed or hemp oil and a tablespoon of ground flaxseed to your cereal before eating.

Lunch

- Khichadi with vegetables
- Upma with vegetables
- Whole-grain pasta with vegetables
- Blissful dal with rice and a side of steamed or sautéed vegetables
- Grilled or baked tofu (marinate with the bliss spice mix) with a bowl of blissful dal

Mid-Afternoon Snack

- 1–2 bliss balls
- 1–2 pieces of fresh fruit such as melon or berries
- Almond milk with spices

Dinner

- Blissful dal with a side of vegetables
- Soup or broth with a side of vegetables
- Smaller portion of khichadi or upma compared to lunch

Note on Vegetables: Steam or sauté vegetables to make them more digestible. Sprinkle the spice mix or fresh herbs with a splash of lemon juice plus olive oil. Another option is to toss cut vegetables with olive oil and spice mix and arrange in a single layer on a baking sheet. Bake at 350°F for 15–20 minutes; if needed, broil at high heat for a few minutes.

A Cautionary Word About Dietary Practices

At this point, I'd like to emphasize that the recommendations made in this chapter don't constitute a "diet." As you have seen, they make up the suggestion to change how you think of food and what that means to your journey to bliss. Some of my patients find these recommendations alarming, particularly if they deviate drastically from what they are used to.

And that is the point—if you are content, blissful, and healthy, you don't need these (or any) recommendations; your lifestyle is working. If not, it isn't working, and perhaps you now have the opportunity to test an alternative. How long must you adhere to these recommendations? The answer is for as long as it takes to get your agni in balance. Perhaps you will arrive at a point when your agni is in perfect balance—when you will be able to eat anything and not be affected. You be the judge.

However, I'd like to caution you against making these (or any) recommendations a religion. Remember the story of Peter, who suffered more by following a "healthy" diet. That is not the point of the Bliss Rx. As a scientist, I don't take anybody's word for anything and prefer to test it for myself. I suggest you do the same. Try out these recommendations and see what works for you in terms of bringing your digestion, senses, mind, and body to balance so that you may discover your true nature. Remember your purpose for doing this program.

The main goal of these suggestions is to enable your body and mind to begin to return to balance so that you can begin your internal housekeeping, which we will see to next.

Summary

- The principles of balancing agni with diet are to regulate neurohormonal pathways and to optimize digestion.

- Balancing vata (the principle of movement) enables the free flow of prana (the subtle essence of vata) through the countless channels of the subtle body.

- A balanced pitta (the principle of transformation) ensures appropriate tejas (the subtle essence of pitta) and that the prana channels don't shrivel up from lack of heat or burn from too much of it.

- Unobstructed flow of prana enables complete digestion and metabolism with the production of ojas, the substance of bliss.

- The diet recommendations of the bliss model take into account the principles of balancing the free flow of vata that is critical for electrical and chemical impulses to travel from cell to cell and from organ to organ.

- The general principles of the bliss diet are to avoid difficult to digest foods, favor simple foods that nourish the body-mind, and follow proper eating etiquette that respects the workings of the pathways.

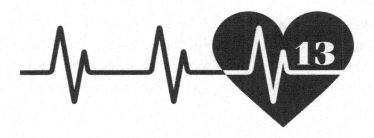

Cultivate Inner Silence

Thus far, we have focused on returning to balance by restoring our neurohormonal pathways through regulating our lifestyles. Now we come to the stage in the program where we turn our attention within. The work we do from here on will focus on the subtle and causal bodies.

Recall that the basis of suffering is a misapprehension of our true nature that arises from the neurohormonal superhighways we have created throughout our lives that have become our habits. Not only do these habits make us do things in certain ways, but they make us think and believe in certain ways that keep us bound to the body-mind as our true identity. They obscure the fact that bliss is our true nature. Let us examine what types of electrical signals in the brain are responsible for this veil that hides us from who we really are.

Brain Waves in Bliss and Stress

If we hooked your brain up with a set of special sensors, we would be able to record its activity and be able to see the following types of electrical activity corresponding to what you are thinking and feeling:

Beta Waves

Ranging from 12–38 Hz (Hertz, a measure of frequency in one cycle per second), we'd see this during most of your waking hours as you engage with the world. When we see beta waves, we see that you are alert, solving problems, making decisions, attentive, and focused. As they get higher in frequency, we would deduce that you are now getting anxious, worried, conflicted, or agitated.

Alpha Waves

We would see these waves ranging from 8–12 Hz if you were very relaxed and still focused. These waves tell us that your thoughts are flowing quietly; you are calm, coordinated, and learning new things or absorbed in something that is of great interest, such as a good book or movie.

Theta Waves

Still slower at 3–8 Hz, theta waves on your brainwave recording tell us that you are either fast asleep or in deep meditation, where you are withdrawn from the world and focused on what you see within. This is also what we'd see when you are about to fall asleep or wake up (the twilight zone, as it is called) and when you are dreaming. This frequency level is where your deepest creativity, fears, troubles, and insights lie, even though you may not be conscious of them. Your sudden "lightbulb" moments come from this frequency. If you can learn to access this frequency consciously, your brain will produce endorphins, those feel-good hormones (chapter 6).

Delta Waves

As we continue to record your brainwave activity, we might come across these ultra-low frequency waves. At 0.5–3 Hz, their appearance tells us that either you are in deep, dreamless sleep or have become detached from the world to revel in your own blissful true nature. This brainwave is deeply healing and restorative, which is why you can fall ill when you don't get enough sleep. It is during the period of this brainwave activity that several beneficial hormones, such as the human growth hormone and melatonin, are released.

Gamma Waves

At 38–42 Hz these brainwaves are the subtlest and highest frequency of all, and if we see this on your tracing, they indicate bliss that radiates to the world in the form of universal love.

By studying brainwaves, we see that each of us has access to all of them. The problem is that the alpha, theta, delta, and gamma waves happen kind of accidentally or in sleep states when we aren't aware of them. The noise of the beta waves keeps the others obscured, since they reside in the realm of silence. In order to access them consciously, we have to cultivate inner silence. Meditation is the tool to cultivate inner silence and reveal the gifts held within.

Numerous studies have indicated that meditation can result in cardiovascular benefit, including the response to stress, smoking cessation, blood pressure reduction, insulin resistance, metabolic syndrome, endothelial function, lack of blood flow to the heart muscle, and prevention of heart disease or additional events after heart attacks. In September 2017 the American Heart Association released a statement that meditation, being a low-cost intervention, could be incorporated along with other lifestyle modifications, with the caveat that larger, more unbiased studies are needed.[39] In the resources section I have listed several organizations where meditation can be learned and practiced. In this chapter I provide the technique that I've used personally and taught for many years.

What Is Meditation?

Despite the seeming explosion of meditation in modern culture, there seems to be a lot of confusion about what it is, being used interchangeably for thinking, daydreaming, or for contemplating a particular issue. With lack of a cohesive understanding about what meditation is, it can naturally lead to confusion about how to practice it and what it is really supposed to do.

---

39 G. L. Levine, R. A. Lange, et al., "Meditation and cardiovascular risk reduction," *J Am Heart Assoc* (28 September 2017), https://doi.org/10.1161/JAHA.117.002218.

Meditation is the precise and systematic technique of allowing the mind to rest in stillness for specific periods of time every day. The purpose of meditation is to dip deep into ourselves to find the bliss that lies hidden under the various states of mind that the brainwaves represent. As we continue to practice, we begin to access the frequencies representing creativity, expansiveness, forgiveness, peace, health, and bliss. Over time, the bliss within begins to radiate outward in the form of universal love, represented by the gamma waves. Before we get into the practice, let us explore some common myths and misunderstandings about meditation:

Myth #1: All meditation techniques are the same.

Response: No. Every technique gives us access to particular brainwaves. There is no one technique that is better than others. It all depends on what we are trying to achieve and how it works for you.

Myth #2: It's enough to meditate once in a while.

Response: Not if we are trying to cultivate inner silence. Just as it is not enough to exercise once in a while to benefit from its positive effects, it takes practice and diligence to cultivate inner silence.

Myth #3: Meditation leads to constant peace and bliss from the get-go.

Response: No. Although meditation will have an immediate calming effect, it often causes friction as it brings up unconscious stuff hidden in our causal bodies. As we gain access to the particular frequencies corresponding to those issues, there can be discomfort in the body-mind, such as irritability, sadness, or anxiety. If this happens, we just scale back on the practice for a few days, knowing that these are actually good signs. We can't work on issues that we can't see, which is the problem with our issues that are hidden from our awareness. When they surface, they invite us to look at them as the cause of our suffering. We can then work through those issues through self-inquiry (see chapter 17).

Myth #4: One doesn't need any other practice; meditation is it.

Response: It depends on what we are aiming for. For stress relief, lowering blood pressure, inflammation and other markers, better sleep, positive outcomes of disease, and a more wholesome perspective on life, meditation is enough. However, these outcomes remain in the default model, where we remain identified as the body-mind. If we want a shift in our identity to the bliss of our true nature, it may not be enough. This is because cultivating inner silence is the key for the advanced practices of self-inquiry and body sensing (chapters 16 and 17), which will not be effective without it. These advanced practices break through our stubborn clinging to our limited body-minds and allow us to realize our true nature. This is why meditation is the central and dominant practice of this program. Balancing agni through a regular routine and lifestyle modifications fosters meditation and vice versa.

Myth #5: Meditation is a religious exercise.

Response: Although there are some faith-based meditation practices, the most prevalent and well-studied ones are secular and universally applicable. The technique you will learn here is from Yoga, which is not a religion but a precise science of our inner landscape. You just have to put the technique to test in your own experience.

Now that we have a definition of meditation, let us see when and how to practice it. The technique I practice and teach in my program is called Deep Meditation and is from Advanced Yoga Practices.[40] I had tried dozens of other techniques before coming across Deep Meditation. Within a very short time of practicing this technique, my life began to change

---

40 Yogani, Advanced Yoga Practices, http://aypsite.com/.

in various ways. The beauty of this technique is its sheer simplicity and applicability. It can be practiced by anyone.[41]

A Note on Children

In general, certain other types of meditation, such as focusing on the breath, is easier and gentler on children because of the issues described under myth #3. A certain degree of emotional maturity is helpful to deal with unconscious issues when they surface, which children may not be capable of. Hence, the recommendation is to wait until puberty to learn Deep Meditation.

When to Practice Meditation

We can use our knowledge about the circadian rhythms to figure out when to meditate (see chapter 11). Recall that vata is dominant in the early hours of the morning until about 6 a.m., and that its subtle actions are more evident on the mind than in the body. It governs creativity, enthusiasm, and cognitive abilities, which peak during vata times. Meditating during this period is thus very effective.

We meditate approximately every twelve hours, in sync with our internal clocks. Meditation resets our functioning at a higher level, which we carry into our daily lives. This higher level of functioning fades over several hours, after which we meditate again. By syncing our practices with our internal clocks, we reset them at a higher level of functioning over time. Thus, we sit again in the evening, preferably before dinner. If this is not possible due to busy evening schedules, my recommendation is to eat early and meditate a few hours later, closer to bedtime. However, don't meditate in bed with the intention of falling asleep immediately after. Meditation is meant to prepare us for activity so that the inner silence we cultivate in the practice is established in daily life. Meditating right before bed can cause sleep disturbances since the body-mind is revved up for activity.

---

41 The Deep Meditation technique is the core practice of my Bliss Meditation Course (kavithamd.com/bliss-meditation-course), which is a free program consisting of various techniques described in this book along with ongoing support.

Even though the best times for meditation are early in the morning and about twelve hours later, keep in mind that it is still highly effective when practiced at any time of the day. So if you can't practice at these preferred times, you will gain the same benefits as long as you practice at all. The most important thing to remember here is to practice with regularity. As long as you fit it into your schedule, you will make great progress.

It is best to meditate on an empty stomach so that the effort of the practice doesn't interfere with digestion. If you're really hungry, a small piece of fruit a half hour before meditation would be okay on occasion. However, try to not make it a habit.

Women can meditate while on their periods. In fact, the mind is much more quiet during the cycle, which enables deeper meditation and greater insights in advanced practices.

As you get established in a daily practice of meditation, continue to apply the principles of regularity and lifestyle that are described in the previous chapters. They will aid the development of a balanced mind and outlook that will in turn help you become established in meditation. The very discipline of meditation will regulate your neurohormonal pathways, which will gently nudge you toward a lifestyle conducive to bliss.

How to Practice Meditation

The Deep Meditation technique is based on mantra. A mantra is a phrase or word that when repeated has the power to transform us from within. The mantra in Deep Meditation is *I Am*, and it is used entirely for its vibratory properties and not for its meaning. The vibrations of the phrase dig deep into our nervous system to rewire our neurohormonal pathways as we access the various brainwaves. Even as it transforms our neurobiology, the mantra pulls us deeper and deeper into the inner recesses of our beings where we come to rest in the bliss and silence of pure awareness. As we get progressively established in inner silence, we naturally begin to wonder about who we really are. The mantra thus facilitates self-inquiry through the cultivation of inner silence.

Here is a breakdown of the practice:

Sitting

The first priority is to make yourself as comfortable as possible to minimize distractions and wanting to shift around. At the same time, your posture must be held gently erect to enable the free flow of prana. So seat yourself either on a chair with a back or on the floor.

Sitting on a Chair: Have both your feet flat on the floor and scooch your back all the way to the back. Let your sit bones ground into the seat, leaving the spine comfortably erect. Your belly is comfortably pulled back to support your spine. Relax your shoulders and place your hands in your lap.

Sitting on the Floor: Sit in any comfortable position. You can try a padded meditation cushion for sitting on the floor. If you are flexible and can easily sit cross-legged or in lotus or half lotus poses, try this pose known as siddhasana (perfected pose) or ardha siddhasana (half of siddhasana). Sit cross-legged on a cushion and bring your left heel under your perineum (the spot between the anus and genitals). If you can, bring your right heel to rest on the pubic bone, the one in the center of the pelvis. This is siddhasana. If you can't or it is too uncomfortable, bend your right leg at the knee and rest it wherever it feels comfortable. This is ardha siddhasana. Often, it helps to have another thin cushion under the tailbone when it becomes comfortable to keep the spine erect. If either of these two poses is too uncomfortable, forget them and sit in an easy pose. In all instances, ground through the sit bones and allow the spine to remain comfortably erect, with your belly supporting it.

Siddhasana (and ardha siddhasana) stimulate the energy center at the base of the spine in the perineum, allowing for the free flow of prana in the subtle body. If you'd like to gain its benefits without the pose, sitting either on the floor or on a chair, you can use a rolled up sock or a soft ball under the perineum and a thin cushion under the tailbone for comfort.

Over time, you will be able to meditate in any posture, even while lying down. For now, however, follow the sitting instructions to get into the practice.

Exercise: Deep Meditation

Close your eyes gently and take a couple of deep breaths, relaxing your body with each exhalation. Notice your stream of thoughts. Now let go of the breath.

Gently introduce the mantra *I Am* by silently thinking it. Listen to its sound by gently focusing on it. When the sound fades, repeat it silently again. Continue to repeat it, waiting for the sound to fade each time. Go at your own pace and rhythm. Especially in the beginning, your attention will drift off into your stream of thoughts and you might start thinking of your grocery list, what you should have said to your friend yesterday, your to-do list for today, a beachside vacation you want to take, and so on. Whenever you realize that your focus is no longer on the sound of the mantra, gently bring it back. Think of it like a baby that keeps spitting out his pacifier and crying to have it back. You gently give it back to him instead of asking him not to cry. Similarly, you favor the mantra instead of trying to force out the other thoughts, which you can never quite do successfully. In this technique, we trick the mind by giving it the mantra as a pacifier to hang on to. Continue this practice for about 15–20 minutes.

When 15–20 minutes are up, keep your eyes closed, let go of the mantra, and rest for about 5–10 minutes. If possible, lie down on your back, using pillows under the head and knees, if needed, for comfort. Let the mind do what it wants to do. Resting is very important in this practice because during deep meditation there is much going on in the subtle body. Whether we feel it or not, there is a sort of scrubbing taking place to loosen and release the deep-seated obstructions that keep us feeling like we are limited body-minds (see myth #3). Resting allows these obstructions to dissolve before we get up and go about our daily life. Resting also allows integration of the inner silence we have just cultivated into the activity we will move on to.

If you begin to experience irritability, restlessness, or discomfort during daily activities, it might be because you are not resting enough after meditation. If you are resting about 10 minutes and are still experiencing these symptoms, it may be a sign that 15–20 minutes of meditation may be too much for you. Try to cut back to 10–15 minutes or even further until you get to a point of feeling good. The reason for the discomfort is that this is a powerful practice that is meant to dislodge the veils that keep us bound to suffering. Ripping these veils all at once is like ripping a tight, sticky bandage off the skin after a wound heals.

Frequently Asked Questions About Meditation

Some questions come up quite frequently when we begin the practice. The following are some of them.[42]

> *Question:* What exactly is inner silence, and how does meditation help cultivate it?
>
> *Response:* The purpose of meditation is to cultivate inner silence. Inner silence is the timeless gap between thoughts, which is available to us throughout the day and frames the doorway to our true nature. Since this is always available, we do not create anything new with meditation; we only become adept at recognizing what already is and has always been. By returning again and again to the object of meditation, the mantra, we cultivate one-pointedness of the mind. The ordinary state of mind is that of diffusion, where multiple and conflicting trains of thought are running at the same time. One-pointedness is the process by which the mind comes to focus on a single object. As we progress, the object becomes increasingly refined to where it is picked up at subtler and subtler levels. The silent gap between repetitions increases, not because the gap is invented (it always is) but because the combination of one-pointedness and refinement leads to its predominance over thoughts.

---

42 Yogani, *Deep Meditation: Pathway to Personal Freedom* (AYP Publishing, 2005).

Question: How long will it take for me to get there?

Response: The most accurate answer is "as long as it will take." There is no timeline for progress in meditation because it is dependent upon our individual makeup of tendencies consisting of our personalities, upbringing, culture, influences, desires, emotional imprints, and repressed and suppressed issues that make up the subtle and causal bodies. In general, the initial results of calmness, reduced stress, health benefits, and sleep regulation occur relatively early, within a few months. The glimpse into our true blissful nature, on the other hand, can take longer, depending upon the particular issues we need to work on through advanced practices like self-inquiry. Technically, however, there is no "there" to get to. As Yogani says, "The journey is from here to here."[43]

Question: I'm not really sure what must happen while meditating. Can you elaborate?

Response: The truth is that every single practice will be unique. While one practice session may be "deep," with relatively fewer thoughts, the next one may be "mind-y," where it feels like no progress was made. It is important to remember that no sitting practice is futile; simply making the time and effort to sit still is a worthwhile endeavor every single time. Meditation works on the neurobiology (consisting not only of the brain and the nervous system but also the subtle and causal bodies) at various levels: at the surface level of thoughts and mind one day and the deeper level the next day. Thus, there is no set thing that "must" happen during any given sitting practice. The beauty of this unpredictability is that it makes us more pliant and forces us to let go of control, an all-important necessity at later stages of spiritual practice.

---

43 Yogani, Advanced Yoga Practices, http://aypsite.com/.

Question: What is the sign of success in meditation?

Response: The only true sign of success in meditation is what happens in daily life. Whether one attains depth in meditation or not is irrelevant if their life is not being transformed because of the practice. This transformation occurs slowly but surely, often first noticed by those around us. Transformation becomes evident in the subtle ways in which we carry ourselves, behave with others, and handle day-to-day matters. Success is noticed when old patterns of reactivity, judgment, and ill will begin to fall away, and we have an increasingly greater capacity to look beyond our narrow selves. It is important to remember that these changes occur whether or not we are achieving perfectly still minds in meditation. Furthermore, achieving a perfectly still mind in meditation is a well-propagated myth. Yes, there are times when this does occur, but this is neither common nor necessary to make progress.

Question: Of all the nuances (posture, timing, duration, and so on), what is the most important factor for progress?

Response: The most important factor is the deliberate cultivation of the habit to meditate. This is the most challenging factor for most of us in the context of already busy lives and overcommitted schedules. It does take effort to make time to practice every day and to adjust our lifestyles to accommodate this. However, this great self-effort is eventually replaced by the meditation taking over the effort and directing itself. This, too, happens without a set timeline. Unfortunately, most people quit before this magical shift occurs. The key is to keep up the practice and have faith that it is working. This applies to any meditation technique: give it enough time (at least a few months) before deeming it a "failure."

Question: What if I don't have 20 minutes to practice? Should I just skip practice that day?

Response: Since cultivating the habit is critical, it is best to meditate for at least a few minutes when short on time. In the same vein, if you are running around and can't sit in your favored spot to meditate, make it a habit to sit for a few minutes elsewhere. Meditate in your parked car before you walk in to work or when you are waiting to pick up your children from school or an activity, in your office before hitting the road, on a park bench before meeting up with friends for dinner, and so on. Be resourceful in finding opportunities so that it becomes a habit, like brushing your teeth.

Question: My mind is so busy during meditation! Does this mean that it is not for me?

Response: This is a common problem for all meditators, particularly when beginning the practice. While we are trying to cultivate inner silence, there seems to be an opposite effect where the mind seems to come alive when we are sitting in practice. Even experienced meditators run into this issue time and again. The reasons for this vary and depend to some extent upon the particular stage of the journey we are in and mostly upon our body-mind makeup with respect to the combination of gunas (sattva, rajas, and tamas). For instance, someone with a predominantly rajasic makeup has an overactive mind streaming with thoughts that run in multiple directions at the same time, while one with a tamasic mind may struggle with laziness during the practice. The good news is that continued meditation practice results in the gradual evolution of gunas, where the mind becomes progressively more sattvic, making it most conducive to deep meditation.

At various stages of the journey, the causes for our mind's agitation may differ; this is completely normal. In the beginning, mental noise may relate to obsessing about the details of the technique, worrying about not doing it right or not being relaxed enough, or thoughts of daily life (the grocery list, dinner plans, the lunch menu, memories of the past, plans for the future, and so on). At later stages, the noise of the surface mind has been quieted enough for the churning of the unconscious mind to become evident. Repressed emotions and trauma, memories of early childhood, and suppressed anger, rage, and anxieties that were deeply hidden from conscious awareness begin to surface. For some, the subconscious mind is active from the get-go, and the jumble of thoughts that come up relate to contents of both the repressed and the surface mind.

Ultimately, however, overanalyzing gunas or the mind's tricks are counterproductive and unnecessary. For our sitting practices to be effective, what we do outside of these practice times can be highly beneficial. As we will see in the next chapter, decluttering our lives takes on a different meaning from the standpoint of enabling meditation and progress along the path to bliss.

Summary

- The various types of electrical activity in our brains correspond to what we are thinking and feeling.

- Generally, the beta waves that correspond to our activities of daily life obscure the beneficial effects of the alpha, theta, delta, and gamma waves that are active at lower degrees of mental noise and reside in the realm of silence.

- Meditation is the tool to cultivate inner silence, which gives us access to these waves.

- Meditation is the precise and systematic technique of allowing the mind to rest in stillness for specific periods of time every day.

- Deep Meditation uses the mantra *I Am* as the tool for accessing inner silence.

- For maximum effectiveness, meditation must be practiced twice a day for 15–20 minutes, followed by resting for 5–10 minutes. In the beginning, cultivating the habit is the most essential piece of the practice.

- If you begin to experience irritability, restlessness, or discomfort during daily activities, it might be because you are not resting enough after meditation. The reason for the discomfort is that meditation can bring hidden issues into our conscious awareness.

- If you are resting about 10 minutes and are still experiencing these symptoms, it may be a sign that 15–20 minutes of meditation may be too much for you. Try to cut back to 10–15 minutes or even further until you get to a point of feeling good.

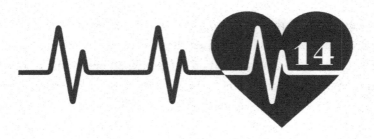

Declutter Your Life

When we take up the practice of meditation, we begin to become acutely aware of our habits, the content of our thoughts, and where we spend our time and effort in daily life. Meditation becomes unpalatable for many of us when the light of awareness shines upon the innumerable things that keep us stuck in suffering. In fact, many people quit practicing because it is far easier to stay stuck than to put in the effort to change our ways. It is a universal human tendency to want to remain in status quo rather than to rise above our limitations, especially when the effort required to change seems almost herculean. The reason for such overwhelm is that our lives and minds are often cluttered.

Driven by the likes and dislikes that make up our neurohormonal superhighways, we become adept at hoarding things in our physical and mental environments. This cluttering of our minds and lives may make meditation difficult, if not impossible, since it is when we are trying to meditate that thoughts of cleaning up arise. We struggle with those thoughts during meditation, but as soon as we get up and go about our day, we are overcome with inertia to clean up!

While many of us focus entirely on the technique of meditation to make progress, the secret to success is to declutter our lives and minds. Think about it. What happens when you post something on social media?

Not only might you eagerly await to see how many likes or comments your post gets, but then you also feel obligated to respond to them. When you are trying to meditate is when the drama comes up, where instead of favoring the mantra, your mind is forming an emotional response to comments or calculating how to word your response without sounding one way or the other. If you have an unfinished project, it will come up in meditation as not only the anxiety of meeting a deadline but also why you hate it or wish you didn't have to do it. If you have a disagreement with someone, guess where the argument will continue? Yes, in your mind while you're trying to meditate. The remedy for these issues is to begin and sustain a serious cleanup project encompassing all areas of your life.

Areas That Need Decluttering

The beauty of this cleanup process is that working on one area spills over into the others. They are interconnected, arising from our minds and projecting to the outside. How we see the world is entirely dependent on our state of mind. When I'm lonely and depressed, the world appears threatening and dangerous. When I'm light and happy, the world appears bright and beautiful. Our state of mind changes our perception. On the other hand, when our environment is clean and beautiful, our state of mind reflects the harmony. Thus, radical decluttering pans across many areas, as described below.

Physical Space

There is something quite magical about a clean, uncluttered space. When we get rid of unwanted stuff there is a shift within that enables us to let go of nonserving thoughts and habits more easily. Before we look at how to deal with the stuff we have, let's examine how we got here. Consumerism is a disease of affluent societies that leads us to acquire things that we don't really need and is driven by the advertisement industry. We are taught to want more and never be content with what we have. One change in a car model is enough to make the previous one undesirable, which is exactly what the car industry is aiming for—to keep you dissatisfied. It is the same story with appliances, gadgets, clothing, cosmetics, and so on. As soon as you buy something, it loses not only its monetary value but also its emotional appeal. You remain dissatisfied and continue to seek contentment in an endless cycle.

Decluttering our homes and physical spaces can become daunting and overwhelming when we don't understand the futility of seeking happiness from elsewhere. This keeps us attached to things that are way past their utility and value, paralyzing us in their hold. Decluttering is a losing proposition when we begin the task of, say, cleaning a drawer and moving the contents to another space. The stuff never leaves; it merely gets rearranged. Since our outer world reflects our inner state, it also indicates our inability to let go of the past and our half-hearted efforts to work on ourselves.

As daunting as it may seem, it helps to declutter your physical space differently. I highly recommend Marie Kondo's *The Life-Changing Magic of Tidying Up*, where the author lays out a simple and effective plan to get rid of unwanted stuff, respect the things you have, and discover the joy and lightness that comes with living and working in a neat, uncluttered space.

Discard or give away everything that isn't useful or doesn't bring you joy. Organize by categories rather than by rooms when decluttering your home so that you are not merely moving stuff from one room to the other. I've found that it is easy to get caught up in sentimentality; I would save every piece of art that my children made and clothing that they had grown out of. Pretty soon we were inundated with their old belongings. When forced to declutter, I had only a few hours and had to make decisions quickly. Moving through the stuff rapidly was the key to effective decluttering, where there was simply no time to ruminate over the baby booties that one child wore just once or a piece of paper with scribbled lines of color from a kindergarten class! With the availability of digital photography, we can now take pictures of the things that are of sentimental value before sending them on their journey elsewhere. Of course, then we are left with the task of organizing photos!

Mind

This is the area where housekeeping can have the biggest impact. Here are the following ways to work on ourselves "off the cushion" so that our meditation practice becomes increasingly effortless and fruitful.

Develop one-pointedness. In a world that is driven by fast-paced multi-tasking, unlearning the habit of doing more than one thing at once is a challenge, but the rewards become amply evident during meditation. Give your complete attention to one task at a time, moving to the next only after it is done to satisfaction. Apply one-pointedness to all areas—turn off the radio and drive in silence, cook in silence, put away the phone while working, pay attention to the conversation when talking with someone, eat in silence and solitude. Make one-pointedness the center of every waking moment; this results in increased efficiency, higher quality of work, greater mental calm, and enhanced creativity.

Complete tasks. Annoyingly enough, it is especially during meditation that thoughts about that incomplete project or the unanswered email surface. Clean up your life's flow by prioritizing and completing daily tasks. Respond to emails and phone calls as soon as possible. Flag or note communications that need to be followed up on. Make technology your obedient servant. If it helps, write down follow-up items and timelines so these details don't clutter the mind. Make it a point to leave no loose ends.

Slow down. Hectic lives such as rushing from one task or appointment to another cannot be particularly conducive to meditation. Wake up earlier and organize your day with enough buffer time between tasks and appointments. At the end of each day, make time to read some inspirational material, even if only for 10–20 minutes.

Cultivate discipline. It is difficult to cultivate a habit for the disciplined practice of meditation if it doesn't extend to other areas of life. Cultivate punctuality, honesty, cleanliness of body and mind, freedom from addictions, and regulated diet, sleep, and exercise habits. Make it a point to sit for meditation every day; forgo a meal (or equivalent) if needed to build discipline. Note that discipline is not the same as obsession, although the line between them can be quite thin. The goal of building a disciplined practice is to test your limits and apply yourself but not to obsess over it. Ultimately, each of us must find a balance between obsession and laxity for all activities, including the discipline and practice of meditation.

Cultivate moderation. Meditation is most conducive when we are neither too full nor famished, when we have had enough sleep (neither too much nor too little), and when we are alert but not agitated. Eat at least 2–3 hours before sitting (which necessarily takes discipline and planning) and practice sleep hygiene.

Let go of likes and dislikes. Our suffering is the result of our attractions and aversions, which form the basis of our neurohormonal superhighways. When we give in to our likes and dislikes, we become enslaved to them, allowing them to dictate how we need to act. Karma Yoga teaches us to do our duty without being swayed by whether we like it or not, and to not get attached to any specific outcome. Think about it—wouldn't our lives be simpler if we just did what we are supposed to do and not do what we are not supposed to do at any given moment?

The challenge, of course, is to know what we are supposed to do and not do at all times. For this, we can call upon our commitments and roles. If you are a parent, you are probably already adept at putting aside your feelings as you do things for your children. You can apply the same attitude toward everything you do, focusing entirely on what needs to be done. Say you have a job that requires you to make decisions about hiring new staff or letting go of some workers. You might hate to be the one to tell someone that their services are no longer required. You might feel guilty about it. However, if you remember what your job calls for, you can focus entirely on what needs to be done. This ability to disengage from the turmoil of emotions is called dispassion, a critical element for progress along the path to bliss.

Dispassion is in direct contradiction to the passion that is so highly prized in the default model. We are taught to be passionate about our goals, which may also include expecting a certain outcome. However, life shows us time and again that the only thing we can be responsible for is our action. The outcome of our effort is never up to us. When we learn to act dispassionately, meditation becomes smoother and deeper as we gain access to unfathomable realms within. Once we give up our likes and dislikes, we step out of their slavery to see everything that lies beyond the box they had created.

Control your senses. Recall that our likes and dislikes are created and propagated through our five senses. Since we take in the world through sight, hearing, smell, touch, and taste, what we take in spurs us into what we put out through the five organs of action—hands in work, legs in motion, speaking apparatus in speech, excretory organs to discard waste, and reproductive organs to produce progeny. If what we take in changes, our actions also change. If we remain enslaved to our senses, we remain entrapped in the neurohormonal pathways that will determine how we behave, which in turn shape our habits, health, and happiness. Examine what you bring in through your senses—what do you see, hear, smell, taste, and touch? What kinds of tastes are you addicted to? Movies, magazines, books, websites? Music, talks, discussions? Are the sense objects that you are chasing serving your purpose of making progress in meditation? If you are a slave to your taste buds and cannot change your eating habits, how can you rewire your pathways? If you are addicted to violent images, how can your actions be nonviolent?

What we take in through the senses comes up not only during meditation but also forms the images of our dreams. It gradually seeps into our subtle and causal bodies, becoming incorporated into our very identities. For Karma Yoga and meditation to be effective, controlling our senses is of paramount importance. Our senses are like wild horses that run amok, wanting this or that, with no ability to decide if it is helpful to our purpose or not. Instead of becoming slaves of our senses, we must regain our mastery over them by holding in the reins and telling them where to go. When we thus control our senses, meditation becomes increasingly effortless.

Learn to surrender. Our minds are such that when we take something away from it, we need to give it something else to hang on to. It is like climbing up a ladder: you let go of the previous rung only when you have a secure footing on the next. When we are learning to let go of our attachment to particular outcomes, it helps to dedicate our actions and their outcomes to a higher ideal. This is called Bhakti Yoga (*bhakti* is love and devotion for a higher ideal).

Devotion is the most essential ingredient for success in any path, but particularly on the journey to bliss. What is devotion? Once again, take the example of parenting where we are utterly devoted to our children. Devotion is guileless love mixed with deep respect, the fuel for commitment. It is devotion to your path that makes you want to continue to tread it.

We can utilize the energy of devotion to cultivate dispassion. Instead of taking ownership for our actions or its results, we devote them to our ideal. An ideal is the image of one who represents perfection to you and can be a religious icon, space, or your own blissful nature, which is absolutely perfect and whole. We are passionate about our actions because we think we are the doer and the enjoyer of their consequences, which is the default model way of thinking. If we get what we want, we feel good, and if we don't, we feel bad. Since we never get what we want every single time, it is a zero-sum game.

In the bliss model, everything in creation moves as a whole and there is no individual doer or enjoyer. Actions are being performed through us, each of us driven by our neurohormonal pathways formed by previous actions. The interaction between you and me is nothing but that of our past actions coming together to create another action. This goes on in an endless cascade of actions and reactions. As we will see in chapter 17, the sense of "I did that" is added on after an action is already in motion.

When we learn to dedicate our actions and their results to our ideal, we stop taking ourselves to be the doer or the enjoyer. This doesn't mean we don't act or don't do a good job. On the contrary, if I am dedicating my action to my ideal, it must be of the highest quality. I humbly offer up my best work as well as whatever comes of it. I stop taking things personally. Detaching from the things of the world is furthered by attaching to our ideal. This approach simplifies our lives in a profound way. When we stop taking things personally, they have nowhere in the subtle or causal bodies to cling to and the neurohormonal superhighways begin to change course. Our meditation practice is strengthened.

Time

Whenever someone says they have no time to meditate, I ask them to list everything they do from the moment they wake up until they fall asleep. Invariably, we find various periods of time during the day where they are being unproductive. Now, unproductive is very different from relaxation or recreation. As we have seen in the previous chapters, relaxation and sleep are critical for our circadian rhythms and to balance agni. Unproductive time refers to time spent in activities that come back to haunt us during meditation. These include time spent browsing the internet; watching the news; discussing politics or current events; posting, commenting, or liking posts on social media; gossiping; attending social functions that are not entirely necessary; talking or texting for no reason; dedication to TV shows or sports channels; and so on. When we cut out unnecessary activities, we suddenly find ourselves with an abundance of time!

Take Jeremy's case, for instance. At sixty-two, he had been meditating for nearly twenty years when he came to see me for a slew of health problems. He had a heart rhythm problem, periodic gout, high blood pressure, and a whole lot of anger. He enrolled in the Heal Your Heart program and found the recommendation for decluttering time to be particularly hard. He was addicted to reading and watching the news and creating stories of catastrophe and doom in his mind. He hung out on the internet with like-minded people that lived in the same shared sense of perpetual threat.

Recall that mirror neurons that enable empathy are also the ones that make us band together in gloom and doom (chapter 6). Add to this the fact that our brains are wired to respond more strongly to negative situations than positive ones—whether they are real or imagined—and we become adept at anticipating the worst in every circumstance. Paradoxically, banding together in gloom harbors attachment (remember oxytocin, the hormone that promotes that yummy feeling of belonging), which is so desirable that it is hard to step out of it.

If progress in meditation is what we desire, we must learn to give up things that do not serve this purpose. Trust that whatever you need to know about current events will make its way to you. Avoid indulging in the news and discussing what is not absolutely needed. Avoid gossip and needless talk. Learn to become quiet inside and out, using the principles of Karma Yoga to speak only when necessary by asking yourself what is needed of your role and commitment at this moment. When Jeremy began to gradually disengage from his way of living, he found himself having a surplus of time to indulge in meaningful activities that didn't cause constant aggravation.

Just as attaching to a higher ideal helps with giving up attachments to our nonserving habits, it is useful to find like-minded people on the same path in order to let go of our need for validation in toxic groups and discussions. However, eventually we will need to stand alone. The path to bliss must be traversed alone, particularly in the advanced stages where the only thing we can rely on is our own wisdom and knowledge. By then, we would have rewired our neurohormonal superhighways and will not require validation from others to feel good about ourselves, and we will have the courage, strength, and beauty to stand in our own blinding light. Until then, judicious use of our precious time is critical, particularly to enable our meditation practice.

Relationships

As you get established in your meditation practice, you will notice that your relationship troubles come up quite frequently to distract you from the mantra in deep meditation. We know now that we are social creatures and thrive on relationships. Close and intimate relationships become our identity, where we start confusing our roles with who we are (see chapter 17). Although relationships enrich our life and bring great beauty and purpose to it, they can become obstructions on our journey to bliss merely because of how we deal with them. Conflict in relationships causes great despair, as each of us knows firsthand. When we don't let go of past hurts, they gnaw at us and come up sooner or later in meditation when the mantra starts shaking stuff out of the causal and subtle bodies. Inner silence cultivated in meditation does heal such wounds. However, it is helpful to facilitate the healing consciously so that meditation becomes more effective.

Make a list of all your relationships, dividing them into essential and nonessential ones. Essential relationships are the ones you have committed to, such as immediate and extended family, those at work and in the community. Essential relationships are ones that mutually nourish each other and keep us grounded. Nonessential ones are those that do not contribute to our lives in any meaningful way, such as those online or on social media (although some of these can be essential), acquaintances, and so on. Which relationships get most of your time and energy? Disentangle emotionally from nonessential relationships by devoting less of your time and energy, not getting involved in the drama, minimizing interaction, and withdrawing from the need for validation.

Resolve conflicts in essential relationships if possible. Take responsibility for your part in the conflict. If the other person doesn't acknowledge it or doesn't take responsibility of their part, understand that this is something they need to work on at their own time and in their own way. Move on. Avoid conflicts in the first place by remaining rooted in your own purpose and path, focusing on any given moment on what you need to do, regardless of whether you like it or not (Karma Yoga). Develop a relationship with a higher ideal and renounce conflicts by surrendering to this wholesome relationship (Bhakti Yoga). Stop taking things personally and see that people behave the way they do because, just like us, they are driven by the neurohormonal pathways they forged in childhood. Perhaps you would have behaved the same way had you formed the same pathways. Who is to say?

As you progress in meditation, the inner silence will work its magic on your perceptions. When this happens, relationships become vehicles of joy and freedom. When it comes to healing from conflicts in relationships and gaining an increasingly blissful perspective, there is no greater tool than self-inquiry, which you will learn in chapter 17.

Self-Doubt and Self-Pity:
Saboteurs of Change

As we go about changing our habits, it is not unusual to be plagued by self-doubt and self-pity. In general, there are two conflicting voices that try to sabotage our efforts: the "naysayer" and the "baby me." You might recognize them when you hear about them. The naysayer is the voice of doubt that wants to keep you entrenched in your old ways. It is the one that wonders if all this is hocus-pocus, if there is really such a thing as bliss, if it is worth all the effort, or if you will ever succeed. You will notice the power of this voice in the following situations:

- Your alarm goes off to indicate that it is time for you to wake up and meditate, and you tell yourself that you'll skip it today.

- You are at a restaurant and can choose between an entrée that you like but know is not conducive to balancing your agni and another that you dislike but know is good for your goal. You pick the first anyway.

- You come face-to-face with someone you've had an undercurrent of conflict with for years. He or she looks at you as if they are about to say hello. You turn around and walk away, allowing the conflict to continue unresolved.

- You are in a work meeting and tasks are assigned for each team member. You dislike your assignment, even though you can carry it out well, and try desperately to switch with someone else.

- You have just quit smoking two weeks ago and meet up with some friends. One of them offers you a cigarette and you think that just one won't hurt, so you accept it.

In each of the above examples, your naysayer voice was hindering your ability to form new habits by instilling you with doubt, laziness, or inertia, where you chose to remain entrapped in your neurohormonal pathways.

The baby me voice works a tad differently but to achieve the same goal. It works through the tactic of self-pity, where you mistake indulgence for self-compassion and self-love. Self-love is not necessarily soft since it stems from wanting the best for ourselves. Think of your children—don't you toughen up and discipline them with the vision of wanting them to fulfill their highest potential? Self-pity, on the other hand, stems from neediness and the sense that you are owed something. It is an overwhelming need to be validated by others and by ourselves. You will notice the power of this voice in the following examples:

- Your alarm goes off in the morning, and instead of waking up to meditate, you tell yourself that you need more sleep since you stayed up watching your favorite show until 1 a.m.

- You are home on a Friday evening and pour yourself a third glass of wine, feeling that you deserve it since you worked so hard all week.

- You are at the water cooler at work when a coworker begins to tell you a juicy story about a mutual colleague. You know you don't want to indulge in gossip but tell yourself you'll do it just this once because you're tired of the office environment and need a break.

- You run into an old flame at a party and find every opportunity to subtly insult him. After all, he deserves it after what he did to you.

In these examples, you can recognize the baby me voice that is trying to keep you glued to your old habits by instilling self-pity, vindictiveness, or a sense of being wronged.

Both the naysayer and the baby me are hurdles to progress, and both beginners and experienced meditation practitioners must learn to deal with them. It helps tremendously to journal extensively, particularly in the beginning. Putting down your thoughts on paper allows you to see what you are dealing with. Once you learn to recognize these voices, you can see that they are simply trying to do their job of keeping you entrapped in your old habits. In fact, these voices arise from the pathways themselves that fear their own annihilation. The identification with the limited body-mind is kept alive by these pathways. Fear of its own demise makes the body-mind churn up stories and strategies to keep you from changing your ways. If you learn to recognize these voices, you will gain mastery over them by learning to ignore them and doing what you are supposed to do to keep you on the path of bliss.

In addition to decluttering our lives, minds, time, and relationships, we can work directly on the subtle body to free up the flow of prana, which can strengthen our meditation practice and enable the cultivation of inner silence. In the next chapter we will see how to do this.

Summary

- The cluttering of our minds and lives makes meditation difficult, if not impossible, since it is when we are trying to meditate that thoughts to clean up arise.

- Declutter your physical space by discarding or giving away everything that doesn't bring you joy or is of absolute use. Organize by categories rather than by rooms when decluttering your home so that you are not merely moving stuff from one room to the other.

- Declutter your mind by developing one-pointedness by completing tasks, slowing down, cultivating discipline and moderation, practicing Karma Yoga through letting go of likes and dislikes and controlling your senses, and practicing Bhakti Yoga by learning to surrender to your higher ideal. Avoid multitasking.

- Use your time judiciously by not engaging in activities that don't serve your purpose.

- Heal your relationships by focusing on essential relationships, resolving and avoiding conflict, and learning to move on.

- Recognize the voices of self-doubt and self-pity that work hard to keep you entrenched in your old nonserving habits.

- Journaling helps tremendously to recognize these voices and gain mastery over them.

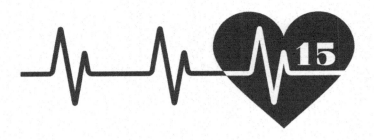

Open to Bliss

Thus far in the Bliss Rx, we have been working on influencing the flow of bliss in our body-mind indirectly by working on our habits, lifestyles, and the mind through meditation. In this chapter we will learn to open to the bliss of our life-force directly. For this we will need to become acquainted with the subtle body, for here is where prana, or life-force, resides.

Recall from chapter 8 that the subtle body is where we take in bits of sensory information from the outside world and process it into meaningful wholes. The subtle body is the animator of the physical body and consists of the following elements:

Subtle Elements of Sense Perception

The elements required for processing sight, sound, taste, touch, and smell are the subtler forms of the great elements. For instance, space is the element required for the processing of sound; without space, there could be no hearing. Similarly, fire is the element for sight, which is why we talk about images being burned in memory. These elements only help with processing information into sensory perception. Based upon our previously formed neurohormonal pathways, we learn to give meaning to sensory perceptions.

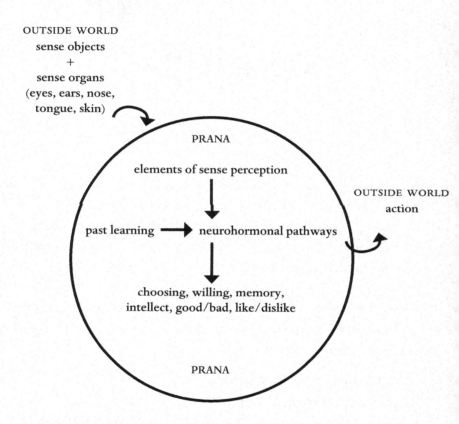

Figure 6: Subtle Elements of Action. Our subtle body (the circle, which represents energy, mind, and intellect) is made up of elements of sense perception, which are dependent on our past learning and determine how we choose our actions.

In other words, the subtle body has the apparatus for converting information from the world into particular experiences. Take the example of a red rose. Your sight apparatus has no ability to see it as a rose. It can only see color and shape. Your conclusions of red, rose, flower, beauty, and so on are based on your past learning. From the perspective of the eyes, the image is registered on the retina, from where the electrical impulses are transmitted to the ophthalmic center of the brain. Nowhere along this path can one find a rose, which is not a function of the sense organs or perception but of the mind, which also resides in the subtle body.

Mind

The faculties of thinking, choosing, and willing belong to what we call the mind. This is where memory of our past gives us our identity as being a specific individual. The mind also displays intellect and wisdom, being able to discriminate between good and bad, beneficial and harmful, and so on. Memory and learning lodged in the mind give us the ability to label sense perceptions; it is because of the mind that we claim to see a red rose. It is also because of the mind with its volitional capability that we can act in specific ways. Will or desire is transformed into action through the organs of action, which also have their roots in the subtle body (see figure 6).

Subtle Elements of Action

Having processed sensory information through the lens of memory and learning, and being driven by the mind's will, we are compelled to act. The compulsion for action encompasses the upper limbs, lower limbs, mouth, genitals, and organs of excretion. Let's return to the example of the red rose. Your organs of perception took in the information. The mind processed it and created the desire to pluck the flower. Your hand reached out to perform the act. These processes are made possible by prana, which is also a component of the subtle body.

Prana

Prana is life force, the fuel for all processes of the body-mind. It is the energy for all of life's functions and flows through fine channels that crisscross throughout the subtle body. Of these, the three most important ones run parallel to the spine, the hot (right) and cold (left) channels flanking a central one. They originate at the end of the spine at the perineum, the left and right channels crossing over to the other side at five locations. At these crossing points the three channels come together, forming wheels of energy known as chakras, which roughly correspond with the nerve plexuses of the body (see figure 7). The side channels end at the nostrils while the center one continues up the back of the head, splitting into two at the midpoint of the brain. One branch continues up to the crown while the other turns straight ahead and ends between the eyebrows. These two points make up the last two chakras. The hot channel crosses over to power the left hemisphere of the brain while the left crosses over to the right.

Not only does the prana running through these channels power the functions of every cell of the body, but it also fuels the workings of the mind. In the body prana is most easily noticed as the vibrations of the breath and switches between the hot and cold channels throughout the day. In the exercise in chapter 8 where you observed your breath patterns, you might have noticed that the right or the left nostril is active at any given time of the day. If you study this switching, you will notice that the dominant nostril will indicate the faculties of the corresponding hemisphere. When the right nostril (left brain hemisphere) is active, you are more likely to be focusing, analyzing, or problem-solving, and your attention is extroverted. On the other hand, when the left nostril (right brain hemisphere) is dominant, your attention is more likely to be introverted, and you might be leaning more toward abstract thinking. The hot channel naturally becomes active when it is time to eat, and the cold when it is time to sleep. Studying your breath rhythms can be highly informative and quite fun!

In the body the two side channels correspond to the sympathetic and parasympathetic nervous systems, with their opposing functions on the organ systems. Importantly, however, the switching of prana from one to the other channel depicts the hallmark of human suffering: duality. We are afflicted by likes/dislikes, attraction/aversion, want/don't want, have/don't have, good/bad, pain/pleasure, and so on. Our lives are marked by the constant seeking of what we like and avoiding what we don't like. Since life doesn't comply with our wishes, we suffer when we get what we don't want or don't get what we want.

If you observe your breath rhythms long enough, you will notice that there are many instances when the breath is even between the two nostrils. If you observe your state of mind when this is happening, you will notice a general sense of peace and contentment. This is because in the process of switching from one side to the other, prana briefly enters the center channel, the channel of bliss. If we can learn to redirect prana to this center channel, we can open to the flow of bliss. This is the purpose of pranayama.

Pranayama

Derived from two words, pranayama (*prana*=life force, *yama*=control) refers to the control of or restraint over the breath. Since the breath is the most visible sign of prana, we can use it to influence the flow of prana. If you are familiar with yoga, you know that there are innumerable pranayama techniques. One way to categorize the techniques would be based on its influence on a particular part of the respiratory cycle. The natural respiratory cycle consists of inhalation, brief pause, exhalation, and brief pause. The various pranayama techniques intervene on one or more of these phases to bring about specific results. For instance, increasing the length of the pause between the breaths is a well-regarded yogic method that supercharges one's neurohormonal system to create new pathways that favor the recognition of bliss. However, such techniques require us to learn from well-accomplished teachers, as the techniques can cause adverse effects when done incorrectly.

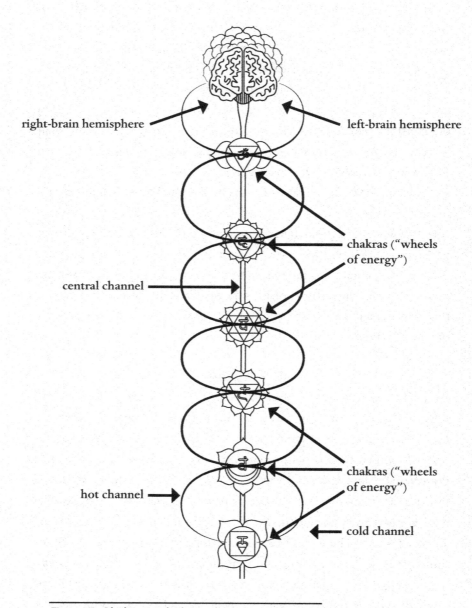

right-brain hemisphere

left-brain hemisphere

chakras ("wheels of energy")

central channel

chakras ("wheels of energy")

hot channel

cold channel

Figure 7: Chakras and Channels. The right (hot) and left (cold) channels flank the central channel that runs along the spine. The two channels cross over at various points along the spine known as chakras (wheels of energy) and end at the opposite brain hemisphere.

While pranayama has shown promise in improving blood pressure and other cardiac risk factors, asthma, cognition, epilepsy, irritable bowel, and other medical conditions, its mechanism of action is not fully known. We do know, however, that its actions are primary on the autonomic nervous system. Recall that unlike the central nervous system, the ANS remains out of our conscious control (chapter 5). Along with the hypothalamus, the ANS regulates all our involuntary body functions through the sympathetic and parasympathetic arms. Although we don't have a direct say in how the ANS works on the body, we can control it through the breath.

Through the deliberate breathing patterns in pranayama, specific stretch receptors in and around the lungs are activated, which carry the impulses to the hypothalamus and the brainstem to increase parasympathetic activity.[44] This action upon the brain results in the rewiring of our neurohormonal pathways, which is an essential component of building resilience to stress.[45]

Resilience is our ability to cope with external stressors (like those we take in from the environment) and internal stressors (like our mind-created worries, anxiety, depression, hostility, and so on). By directly manipulating our levels of oxygen and carbon dioxide in the blood, we influence the activation of the brain centers to build new pathways by changing the electrical and chemical signaling within cells.

In pranayama we restrain the breath just enough to create a vacuum-like effect in the nervous system, where prana rushes in from the subtle body to fill the space. It starts moving through channels that were previously obstructed by the other components of the subtle body—the mind and elements of perception and action. This is much like turning on the water after a prolonged period of disuse, when the pipes have collected dirt and residue. The flow of prana begins to dislodge our misperceptions

---

44 R. Jerath, J. W. Edry, V. A. Barnes, and V. Jerath, "Physiology of long pranayamic breathing: neural respiratory elements may provide a mechanism that explains how slow deep breathing shifts the autonomic nervous system," *Med Hypotheses* 67 (2006): 566–71.

45 K. S. Carter and R. Carter, "Breath-based meditation: A mechanism to restore the physiological and cognitive reserves for optimal human performance," *World J Clin Cases* 4 (2016): 99–102.

about the world and ourselves, cleansing us from deep within. The wheels of energy that were previously stagnant or sputtering begin to gain momentum and whirl with life. We notice these effects gradually as the entire way in which we perceive life begins to change, becoming increasingly saturated with bliss.

When to Practice Pranayama

With continued practice, the vacillation between the two side channels decreases as the ANS is brought more into balance. With equilibration between the two channels and the two hemispheres of the brain, prana begins to make its way up the center channel. Prana gathering in the center channel naturally evokes inner silence, the perfect state for meditation and higher practices. This is why we practice pranayama directly before meditation.

Practice pranayama for 5–10 minutes before meditation with no break between the practices. Rest after meditation for 5–10 minutes. If you are running short on time and can only fit in one practice, meditation takes precedence. However, you will notice quickly that adding a few minutes of pranayama right before meditation changes the dynamic of the mantra.

How to Practice Pranayama

Before we delve into a simple pranayama technique, I invite you to pause for a moment and observe your breath without changing it. Which part of your torso is moving with breath? Is your belly moving in or out with the in-breath? What does it do with the out-breath? If you're like most people, most of your breathing involves the top portions of the lungs and your belly moves in with the in-breath and out with the out-breath. If you get a chance, observe a sleeping baby. You will see the opposite rhythm, where her belly moves out with the in-breath and in with the out-breath. This is the natural, spontaneous rhythm of the body that enables the lower part of the lungs to participate in breathing.

When you breathe in, your belly should inflate, which creates a sucking effect on the diaphragm so it is pulled down. When you breathe out, your belly should move toward the spine, which pushes the diaphragm up to aid the exhalation process. Check your breathing as you go about your day and revert to abdominal breathing if needed. This will help you in your pranayama practice.

Exercise: Pranayama

Sitting: Follow the sitting instructions for meditation (chapter 13). Sitting in siddhasana or ardha siddhasana helps activate the channels of energy in the perineum. Alternatively, you can use a rolled-up sock or ball under the perineum for the same effect.

Beginning the Practice: Close your eyes gently and take a couple of deep breaths, relaxing your body with each exhalation.

Hand Position: For this practice of alternate nostril breathing, you will use your dominant hand. If using the right hand, use the thumb to close your right nostril and the ring and pinkie fingers to close the left (if you can't, use the middle finger).

The Main Practice: Close your right nostril as you breathe out and then breathe in through the left. Close the left nostril and breathe out through the right. Breathe in through the right, close the right nostril, and breathe out through the left.

Each in-breath and out-breath is slow, deep, and deliberate, your belly moving out with the in-breath and moving in with the out-breath. Allow your chest to expand fully with each in-breath and exhale fully as it contracts. Try to roughly equalize the duration of your in-breath and out-breath. At the end of 5–10 minutes, rest your hand in your lap and begin deep meditation.

Lessons Learned from Pranayama

As we learn to reap the benefits of restraining the breath, the wisdom of this approach spills over into all the areas of our lives in the form of discipline. These benefits are subtle and cannot be reliably measured since they are subjective. We begin to learn that controlling our senses, habits, and lifestyles in particular ways leads to benefits in other ways. If I can resist the temptation to indulge in sweets, I will enjoy the benefits of hormonal balance and good health. If I can resist the temptation to buy things that I don't really need, I will have to work less. If I can resist the temptation to fall back asleep when my alarm goes off, I will progress faster on the path to bliss.

Pranayama and meditation enhance each other in that the restraining discipline of pranayama teaches us to gently favor the mantra in meditation when other thoughts may seem more seductive. The stillness cultivated through meditation enables the free flow of prana and makes pranayama stable. The combination of the two practices enables us to focus on deeper levels of silence until the mind becomes completely still to reveal underlying bliss.

Summary

- The subtle body is where we take in bits of sensory information from the outside world and process it into meaningful wholes. It consists of the subtle elements of the organs of perception and action, the mind, and prana.

- The elements required for the processing of sight, sound, taste, touch, and smell enable the registration of sensory input.

- The faculties of thinking, choosing, and willing belong to what we call the mind. This is where memory of our past gives us our identity as being a specific individual.

- The compulsion for action flows out from the subtle body to the upper limbs, lower limbs, mouth, genitals, and organs of excretion as a response to registering information gathered via the sense organs.

- Prana, the energy for all of life's functions, flows through fine channels that crisscross throughout the subtle body. Of these, the three most important ones run parallel to the spine, the hot (right) and cold (left) channels flanking a central one.

- Switching prana from one channel to the other depicts duality, the hallmark of human suffering.

- Derived from two words, pranayama (*prana*=life force, *yama*=control) refers to the control of or restraint over the breath.

- In pranayama we restrain the breath just enough to create a vacuum-like effect in the nervous system, where prana begins to flow through channels that were previously obstructed by the other components of the subtle body—the mind and elements of perception and action.

- Pranayama is best practiced right before meditation, where the two practices enhance each other.

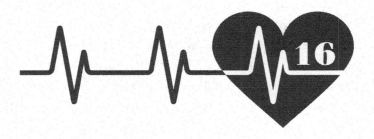

Cultivate Clarity
of Perception

Imagine this scenario: you walk into the conference room at work where three of your coworkers are talking in whispers. As soon as you step into the room, they stop talking and take their seats. What is your first thought? How do you respond to them as your meeting progresses?

The way we respond to everyday occurrences is entirely colored by our perception, which in turn is determined by our neurohormonal superhighways. We interpret our experiences not only according to our inner state, but we also take them very personally. Quite simply, we feel strongly that the world is out to get us. In every interaction, our immediate thought is what it may mean for us. Think about how you interpret the news—whether it is about a hike in taxes, a local crime, or a natural disaster, your first thought is about how it affects you. This isn't a personality flaw or an issue with any one of us in particular. It is the way we are wired, thanks to the pathways we build in response to our upbringing and learning. Not only do we immediately jump to (usually wrong) conclusions, but we hold them to be true.

In the above scenario, your first thought might have been that your coworkers were talking about you behind your back, when they might have been discussing an issue that was completely unrelated to you. If you felt that your colleagues were talking about you, your future interactions with them will be colored by the incident. See how we propagate suffering?

To live a life of joy and fulfillment, we must learn to clean the lens through which we view the world and interpret our experiences. This is the purpose of self-inquiry, a powerful tool for inner housekeeping. In this chapter we will explore the concepts that keep us bound to suffering and make it hard for us to experience true compassion, forgiveness, acceptance, and love.

Of all the components of the Bliss Rx, self-inquiry is the subtlest and therefore the most challenging. It takes a deep interest in becoming free of suffering to sustain the practice, along with ongoing deep meditation. With repeated practice, self-inquiry opens us to immense joy and sweetness by peeling away all that obscures our true identity, eternal bliss consciousness.

A Closer Look at Suffering

So far in this book, we have looked at the way our neurohormonal pathways are formed from a biological standpoint. Let us now look at the basic constructs of suffering from a psychic perspective, connecting it back to the neurohormonal superhighways. What is it that makes us jump to conclusions and trigger the cascade of reactions?

Assigning Truth to Experience

For us to react to a situation, we must first assign an element of truth to our experience. In the above example, your immediate reaction that your coworkers were talking about you might arise from a past experience where you might have felt excluded in a peer group or discovered that somebody was indeed talking about you. The conclusion you reached at the time (which is now unconscious) is that people generally exclude you or talk about you behind your back. Of course, your rational mind may know that this is not true. However, as long as you react to a situation, you can be assured that it is your subconscious mind that is in control and not your rational mind. And reactions occur because, at some level, you believe this to be true.

Simply believing that something is true doesn't cause all the pain and grief. Not only do we assign truth to our experiences, but we also believe that they should be different. You don't suffer because you believe that your coworkers talk behind your back. You suffer because you believe that they should not behave this way. If you did not have the ability to believe such a thing, it would make no difference to you whether they talk behind your back or not. Wanting things to be different than they are is what causes much of our suffering.

Taking Thoughts Seriously

Notice that you have no control over your thoughts. You can't choose what thought is going to come up next. From the standpoint of the mind, thoughts are just wave forms that arise and subside mostly randomly. In fact, 95 percent of our thoughts are useless autobiographical ruminations that arise from the default mode network (chapter 7). Only 5 percent of our thoughts are directed toward tasks at hand, planning, and other useful functions. If we can see that thoughts just come and go and not take their content seriously, our lives would improve instantly.

Not Taking Responsibility for Our Experience

Ponder this for a moment: everything we do is based on wanting to feel a certain way. Every choice we make, every interaction we have, and every reaction that arises has its roots in our limbic system–driven neurohormonal pathways and the hormones that make us feel good or bad. In early life we learn what feels good and what doesn't, and this becomes the lens through which we view everything that comes our way. We take things personally when every situation is completely neutral. How I interact with you has absolutely nothing to do with you and everything to do with my own lens. My happiness (or lack thereof) is entirely a product of my lens. No circumstance, situation, or person is responsible for my happiness or peace. In other words, our experience of life is entirely dependent upon the lens through which we view it. The mind can be our best friend or our worst enemy.

Taking Our Mental States to Be Who We Are

Taking our stories to be who we are is the root cause of our suffering. Recall that our neurohormonal pathways are forged in early childhood and are based entirely on our life experiences and what we are taught about ourselves. We learn who we are based on what our caregivers tell us, such as "I'm good in math, I have pretty hair, I'm not a good singer," and so on. These impressions and thoughts become the labels that define us. In adolescence the labels become more complex, such as "I'm unlovable, I'm not as good as my peers, I'm shy, I'm an extrovert," and so on. As we age, we add more labels to define ourselves based on our life experiences: "I hate people who whine, I love selfless people, I'm a pretty good citizen, I'm a Republican, I'm a cancer survivor, I have joint pains, I'm anxious," and so on. What we call I is nothing but a mish-mash of stories, thoughts, feelings, and beliefs. And this misapprehension is a result of judging a situation according to our definition of truth and how it should be different. We take the "should" thoughts seriously because we are unable to see that our reaction to the situation is merely the product of our lens. Our judgments form our I and thrive on validation and justification.

Validating and Justifying the I

Stop for a moment and contemplate why you do what you do. How many times a day do you think to yourself why you "need" something? What happens when you send a thoughtfully composed email and don't receive an acknowledgment? The bottom line for why we do what we do is that we are constantly seeking validation from others for our experience, and this need for validation is supported by justifying our actions to others and to ourselves. I "need" a third cup of coffee because "I'm used to it and I can't function without it," and so on, each need based on how I define myself. Having a third cup of coffee defines who I am, and so I justify my need for it. If I don't have the coffee and get a headache, it validates my label of being the one who needs it. See? So we go about our lives justifying our actions based on who we think we are and seeking validation to make it seem true. If you validate my choices and actions, my sense of I is fortified and I like you. If you don't, I get upset and dislike you. Seeking approval and validation from others (and ourselves) is the only way this false sense of I is kept alive.

Witnessing: The Prelude to Self-Inquiry

In order to be free of suffering, we need to be able to look at our thoughts and beliefs in a nonjudgmental fashion. This is known as witnessing, where we stand apart from our experience and simply watch it as it unfolds. The most effective way to cultivate witnessing is through meditation. When we can watch the mantra as it arises and subsides, we notice that we can watch our thoughts and actions. The following practice helps with the deepening of witnessing. Do this practice every evening, preferably after your meditation and just before resting. Alternatively, you can practice this technique before bed.

- Play your day like a movie in your mind. How did the day's events unfold? What were your thoughts about as you went through your day? When you were interacting with others, what were you thinking about? What could you have done differently?

- As you recall your day's experience, notice the thoughts and feelings that come up in the present time. Do you feel satisfied, regretful, sad, angry, lonely, hopeful? Watch these thoughts as they come up, knowing that they are just thoughts and feelings arising from your neurohormonal superhighways. Can you watch them without becoming pulled into their stories?

- End the practice after 5–10 minutes by lying down and resting.

As you become adept at observing your mental processes without becoming entangled in them, you'll be able to notice your thoughts as they arise in daily life. This phase of this path is a key turning point, when self-inquiry can begin to make the most difference. Unless we can disengage from our mental processes, we cannot effectively inquire into them.

You must be able to see your mind's activity like a movie and know that it *is* a movie!

Once you are able to stand apart from your thoughts, you can delve deep into the following self-inquiry practices. Here we will inquire into each aspect of suffering as we defined it above.

Assigning Truth to Experience

Byron Katie's book *Loving What Is* is based on inquiring into the presumed truth of our experience. A superbly effective self-inquiry practice, I recommend this book and technique known as "the Work" to anybody who is interested in loss of suffering. In this practice we examine our beliefs and thoughts in a unique fashion using four questions.

Say, for instance, that I have a gripe with Fred, who, in my opinion, does not treat others kindly. This bugs me. So I work with this situation in the following way.

I notice the thought that says "Fred should be kind." This thought causes me stress because I see that Fred is not behaving appropriately, and I think he should be. The first question I ask myself is, "Is this true?" Do I know with certainty that Fred should be kind? The brutally honest answer is that I don't know what Fred *should* be doing with absolute certainty. When I think about it some more, I find that I'm not absolutely certain that kindness looks a particular way.

Next I ask myself whether this thought causes me peace or stress. It causes stress because I'm trying to dictate Fred's actions, which only he has control over. The only truth of the experience is that Fred behaves the way he does. When I try to change reality to be other than what it is, I suffer. Reality doesn't change because I think it should be otherwise. It will always be as it is. In this inquiry, then, I suddenly realize that the source of stress is not Fred's behavior but my thought that it should be different.

Then I wonder who I would be without this thought. When I sit quietly with this, the silence within shows me that without this dictatorial thought, I am at peace.

Finally, the Work asks us to do the turnaround, which is to find an opposite statement that is equally true. Here, one turnaround may be "Fred should not be kind." This is equally true because he isn't kind according to my definition. Another turnaround is "I should be kind." This statement is even truer considering the violent nature of my judgmental thoughts about him. The important thing to realize is that whatever we don't like in others arises because we possess the same quality within ourselves. What is really bothering me about Fred is that I am unkind, and it is easier for me to project it onto him than to look at my own process.

With this inquiry I come to see my business versus Fred's. When I stay in my business, I'm at peace. When I meddle with Fred's (or anyone else's) business with my shoulds and should nots, I suffer. So I choose to stay in my business, allowing things to be as they are and working on my own thought processes.

Exercise: **Assigning Truth to Experience**

Here is one way you can practice this form of self-inquiry:

- Recall a situation that causes you discomfort. It might be an interaction you had with someone, an outcome you did not expect, a world event that is frightening, or an anticipated situation that makes you anxious.

- Notice your thoughts about the person or situation—is your discomfort arising from them or your judgment about them? Judgments arise as "should" and "should not" clauses.

- Who would you be in this moment without the stories that fuel the judgments?

- Can you find a turnaround for your situation? Can you see what it is in yourself that you are projecting onto the person or situation?

Taking Thoughts Seriously

While questioning the truth of our experience is a critical step in the process of self-inquiry, it is only the beginning. Many of us can continue to take arising thoughts to have inherent meaning. Our clever minds can devise ways to continue believing in some thoughts and question only those that cause discomfort. In this all-too-common situation we tread the thin edge of suffering and can fall off the cliff at the slightest provocation. The key to freedom from the tyranny of thoughts is to see that they are arisings in our awareness and that they come and go without voluntary control.

For effective inquiry into thoughts, it helps to understand the difference between arisings and awareness. Greg Goode's *The Direct Path: A User Guide* is a fantastic resource for inquiry into our experience, including thoughts. The preparatory exercise for this type of inquiry is called the heart opener, and I recommend this practice highly.

Exercise: The Heart Opener

- Close your eyes and take a few slow and deep breaths. Relax.

- Notice that sensations in your body, noises and other sensory stimuli, and thoughts and feelings come and go, but you are always present here now.

- Whether or not sensations, thoughts, and feelings occur, you are always present here now.

- When sensations, thoughts, and feelings are present, you know that they are present. When they are absent, you know that they are absent. You are always present, whether or not these objects arise.

- You are the awareness in which all objects arise and subside.

- Notice if there are borders to this awareness. If the sense of a border comes up, notice that this sensation is yet another object that arises in you, which is awareness. You (awareness) are without definition, border, or limit.

- All descriptions of awareness (clarity, space, vastness, and so on) arise as objects in awareness.

- Return to this exercise before each session of inquiry (or even during inquiry if you find yourself caught up in the mind). Take a few minutes every day to sit with this exercise at the end of your meditation.

An innocent mistake we tend to make is to try to "find" awareness or want to experience it. However, awareness is the sole subject of all experience. Anything that we find in it is an object, including all experiences, sensations, and thoughts. Awareness cannot be known or found as an experience because it is what knows. Awareness doesn't say yes to a pleasant experience and no to an unpleasant one. Even our darkest thoughts, experiences, and feelings are welcomed into awareness with sweetness and love. This practice is called the heart opener because of this inherent sweetness that it evokes.

The heart opener can initially feel difficult and forced, and we can keep getting caught up in the objects arising in awareness. This is natural. As we practice, we will come to see that the mind is itself an object that arises in awareness.

Let's now take the example of memory and examine thought closely.

- Begin with the heart opener exercise.

- Recall what you had for lunch yesterday. Bring up the memory as vividly as possible, including the taste, smell, and sight of the food. Take your time.

- You're recalling the thought of a meal, but is the meal really here? What is this thought arising as in your awareness?

- Now examine another thought about the weather today. What is this thought arising as in your awareness?

- Is there a difference between the thought of your meal from yesterday and that of the weather today? To awareness, both are just arisings.

- In your direct experience while taking a stand as awareness, do either of these thoughts have any assigned truth to them? What does the experience of truth arise as?

Let's break down this inquiry. You had the experience of the meal yesterday, which was a group of sensations arising in your awareness: the smell, taste, and sight of the food, of feeling full, and so on. Today when you think of it, it is a group of thoughts arising in awareness—the *memory* of the smell, taste, and sight of the food, how it made you feel, and so on. All sensations and thoughts come and go. You, the common denominator as awareness, are always here now. The memory of yesterday is arising as a thought here now.

When you examine thoughts about the weather, they too occur as arisings in awareness here now. To awareness (you), thoughts about yesterday, tomorrow, or today are all the same arisings. Let's see how a thought appears to make sense or feel like truth.

- Your thought about the weather came up: "It is hot today." To awareness, this thought is no different than a thought saying "blah, blah."

- This was followed by another thought that validated the first thought to be true.

We take thoughts seriously because thought says it is true, not because there is inherent truth to thought. Examine your biases and beliefs closely and you will see that all thoughts are mere arisings in awareness—they come and go. If we learn to take a stand as awareness rather than as a mass of thoughts, we lose the ability to take thoughts seriously.

Taking Responsibility for Experience

The main reason that we suffer in relating to the world is because we think that the world is "out there" in contrast to the self that is "in here." However, standing as awareness shows us that everything in our experience is always occurring "in here" and that there is nothing "out there." You've probably heard the story of a group of blind men that encountered an elephant. Each person feels a different part of the elephant and comes to a different conclusion—the one touching the trunk calls it a rope, the one touching the limb calls it a tree trunk, and so on. Similarly, you and I would interpret an object, behavior, or situation differently based on our particular neurohormonal pathways. Neither of us would be absolutely right or wrong. However, both of us would be wrong to assign objectivity to experience, which is always subjective.

To be completely objective, we would have to step out of awareness and "look in." Could we ever step out of awareness? Where would we go? Wherever we go, we are always "here" in awareness. Whatever we see, hear, touch, smell, and feel is in awareness.

Let's examine this principle with a simple exercise. For this, let us use an object you use in daily life, such as a cereal bowl. Keep the bowl at eye level where you can see it clearly.

- Begin with the heart opener exercise.
- Look at the bowl. Take in the color, pattern (if any), shape, size, and any other characteristics that catch your eye.
- Without the label of "bowl," what do you see?
- Now tune in to the sensation of seeing. Is there a boundary between seeing and the bowl? Is there somewhere that seeing ends and the bowl begins?
- You are aware of seeing. Is there a boundary between awareness (knowing that you are seeing) and seeing itself? Is there somewhere where awareness ends and seeing begins?

In this exercise we see that the function of seeing is only capable of perceiving color and shape. Seeing cannot see a bowl, which is a label given by learning. Patterns and depth are deduced by shades of color and contrast between the bowl and the surroundings.

There is no separation between seeing and color. There is no unseen color; the only way to verify color is to see it—you can't smell it, taste it, hear it, or touch it. Color implies seeing. There is no point in our direct experience where seeing ends and the color begins.

Further, there is no separation between seeing and awareness. As soon as you say "I see," you are implying that you know that seeing is happening. In your direct experience, then, color arises in awareness as awareness, just as the wave arises in the ocean as the ocean. If you observe all of your senses, you will come to the same conclusion: sound is not separate from hearing and hearing is not separate from awareness, odor is not separate from smelling and smelling is not separate from awareness, touch is not separate from feeling and feeling is not separate from awareness, and taste is not separate from tasting and tasting is not separate from awareness.

This discovery leads to a sense of relief and wonder. When you see that the way you sense the world is not separate from your awareness, your relationship with the world changes. There is no separation between you and the world. It is all occurring in you; there is nothing outside of you. When you extend this observation to your inner processes, you see that your thoughts, emotions, memories, and moods also are never separate from awareness. You are that in which all these arise and fall—you are the knower of all states, sensations, thoughts, and emotions. Like the movie screen that remains untouched and pristine whether the movie is a romantic comedy or a scary horror flick, you, awareness, remain unaffected and blissfully aware. All characters occur in you. It is only because you forget that you are the screen that you suffer.

How do you experience another person? Through your senses, of course. You see, touch, smell, hear, and feel them. Whether the sensations evoke attraction or aversion in you has nothing to do with them and everything to do with you and your conditioning created by your neurohormonal superhighways. Based on your conditioning, you decide whether you like them or hate them, whether they are worthy or unworthy, whether they can be trusted or not, and so on. Your judgments are also arising in awareness. Thus, the person is arising in your awareness, and your judgment about them is arising in awareness. There is nowhere else that they can arise.

To take responsibility for our experience is to own that nothing and nobody is responsible for our circumstances, thoughts, and actions except ourselves. We stop viewing ourselves as victims in this great understanding, the result of which is total forgiveness of others and harmony with the world.

Mistaking Moods and States for Identity

Once you get the hang of standing as awareness, you will realize that there is no such thing as objectivity. Despite this understanding, there can be a subtle identification with our moods and states, taking them to be who we are. Once again, we can investigate our darkest moods and our greatest ecstasies to see if that is who we are.

Think of a pink elephant. Where was this thought a moment ago? Was it hiding somewhere and surfaced into your awareness? Examination of direct experience shows us that the thought of a pink elephant arose in awareness, lasted for a while, and subsided back into it. One analogy for this is the ocean and its waves. Are waves hiding somewhere outside of the ocean and jump in to manifest? No. They arise out of the ocean and subside back into it. Similarly, sensations, thoughts, emotions, and moods arise and subside in awareness.

Awareness is knowingness. To be aware is to know experience as it arises. As you read this, your focus might be on the words on the paper. However, notice that we can read or see words entirely because of the white of the paper in the background. Similarly, awareness is the light of knowingness of all states and moods. Knowing is neutral and without judgment. It is the suchness or is-ness or being-ness of experience. Can there be an experience of objects (and here we define every arising as an object, be it a physical, mental, emotional, psychological, or other experience) without awareness of them?

Take a bad mood, for instance. It arises in awareness, stays for a while, and subsides back into it. You are always present. How can you be your mood if you don't come and go with it? Similarly, ecstasy, joy, and pain arise and subside in you, awareness. The classic teaching in Vedanta is to see that whatever you think you are is not you since all thoughts and beliefs about who you think you are are objects arising in you, awareness. You, awareness, are the subject. Objects come and go, but you, as awareness, are eternal, untarnished, and ever blissful.

Validating and Justifying the I

If you become vigilant and critically observant of your thoughts, you will notice how your neurohormonal superhighways reinforce themselves through constant validation and justification. Even as you read this, your superhighways are being reinforced by agreeing or disagreeing based on your previous experiences but mostly based on what it means for your I. We are inherently self-absorbed and self-centered simply because of the way we are wired. Just as we had innocently taken our subjective experience to refer to objectivity, we are programmed to keep our individual I alive to facilitate our primal instincts of survival and reproduction (see chapter 7).

The mystery of the I is that it is shaky and unreliable. Ordinarily, we define the I to be made up of likes and dislikes, the roles we play, our life histories, and so on. If my life history was one of struggle and disappointment, I will interpret all my situations to reflect how I got through it. If I'm ridden with resistance to struggle and my idea of an ideal life is one of no struggle at all, my I is one that is always disappointed or unlucky. In everything I do, I validate the I, unconsciously finding struggle. In an innocently twisted way, finding situations difficult satisfies my belief of what my I is. If, for instance, I put in a lot of work on a project and don't get the credit I deserve, my I is validated through my history of struggle with thoughts such as "This always happens to me. No matter what I do, I never get credit. I've been dealt a bad hand by fate," and so on. Even having a serious illness can become a way to validate the I, with the suffering acting as an anchor for who we take ourselves to be.

Each of us is always seeking validation for being who we think we are. When we are not seeking validation, we are justifying the I with explanations to ourselves or others about why we need/don't need, want/ don't want, or like/don't like something. Notice the constant drone of the voice in your head that is veering you toward seeking validation or justifying your actions. Why do you agree to take on a project? How does it validate you? How do you justify your waking up late, having another cup of coffee, choosing a meal or clothing or one course of action over another? Notice that all the choices we make are based on validating or justifying the I. Is there really freedom in our choices if we are bound by our neurohormonal superhighways to feel validated or justified?

The antidote to validation and justification is to see the true nature of the I as a collection of memories and labels that create a story. Who are you without your story? We can investigate this with the following exercise.

Exercise: Who Are You?

- Begin with the heart opener exercise.

- How do you define yourself? Write it down, if it helps. Notice that every definition of your I is an object arising in awareness—thoughts about your roles, memories, being a particular gender of a particular nationality or race, having a disease, being happy, sad, serious, shy, creative, introvert, extrovert, worthy, unworthy, loving, unloved, secure, insecure, and so on. They arise and subside, but you, awareness, are always present. How can these labels be you if they come and go?

- As you go about your day, observe your thoughts as they arise to validate or justify your sense of I. Notice that they arise from habit but don't really define who you are.

- Journaling is very powerful in this exercise. Become totally honest and transparent as you write down all the subtle ways in which you seek validation—where your I wishes to be seen.

As we learn to take a stand as awareness, the stories we tell ourselves about who we are begin to disintegrate. We gradually come to see that we are not our stories and that who we are is open, ever-loving, and blissful awareness in which the stories come and go.

Self-inquiry is the scalpel that digs up and excises the tumor of suffering. Through the various practices in this chapter, we come to see the root cause of suffering, which is identification with the body-mind. Through self-inquiry we question our most treasured beliefs and truths that subtly bind us to suffering. Questioning them opens us to the light of our true identity of bliss, resulting in a paradigm shift. Then we see that who we are is never separate from all of creation.

When we start delving into self-inquiry, it is common to mix up two different levels of experience: the relative and the absolute. For instance, discovering that no two thoughts are related can cause confusion—how can we sustain our lives if there is no continuity in our relationships or interactions? This is the predicament of mixing up levels. On an absolute level and from the standpoint of awareness, there are no two related thoughts. Paradoxically, when this truth becomes well-established in our experience, we open to great joy and freedom on the relative level. We can have intimacy in interactions and relationships because our heart is wide open to all possibilities.

Thus, it is best to try to not mix up the absolute and relative levels. We can continue to live our lives and simultaneously inquire into our experience. Soon, the seeming contradiction between them will dissolve into blissfulness in our daily lives. Awareness is all there is—blissful, eternal, and ever-pure. This paradigm shift opens us to a sweetness of being where we remain engaged in the world like before, but whereas in the past there was a sense of separation and pain, we are now in unity and wholeness with all. In this joyful model we stop taking our stories seriously because we have seen through them. This is the end of suffering.

Summary

- To live a life of joy and fulfillment, we must learn to clean the lens through which we view the world and interpret our experiences. This is the purpose of self-inquiry.

- When we assign truth to experience, we suffer from wanting it to be different.

- If we can see that thoughts just come and go and not take their content seriously, our lives would improve instantly.

- Our experience of life is entirely dependent upon the lens (neurohormonal pathways) through which we view it. There is no objectivity to experience.

- Taking our stories to be who we are is the root cause of our suffering.

- Validating and justifying the stories of who we think we are keep us bound in the quagmire of suffering.

- Through self-inquiry we come to question our most treasured beliefs and truths, which opens us to the light of our true identity of bliss.

- In this joyful new model we stop taking our stories seriously because we have seen through them. This is the end of suffering.

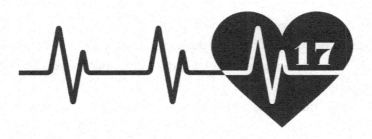

Find Bliss in the Body

Once we become familiar with the exercises in the previous chapter, we can begin to work on the aspect of ourselves that feels so true and solid that it keeps us in a perpetual state of tension and contraction: the body.

Pause for a moment to answer this question: How do you know your body? When you go to sleep at night, the body disappears. When you wake up in the morning, it reappears. What does it reappear as? Ordinarily, we would say that we experience the body as a solid mass of flesh and bones subject to health and decay. You might think of your body as having a certain mass, shape, coloring, and size, with particular characteristics, such as the shape of your nose, the contour of your belly, buttocks, or breasts, and so on. You might also associate it with specific health issues, such as stiff joints, heart disease, or cancer. In other words, you know your body through an image and collection of sensations. The image we have of our bodies becomes crystallized through constant reinforcement via the neurohormonal superhighways.

You look in the mirror every morning and carry the memory of the image of your body, becoming self-conscious or self-confident based on what you think it should look like. Over time, this image becomes so embedded in your psyche that you start taking the image to be your body. When the image suffers, you suffer. If your idealized image of the body is one that is of a particular size, shape, and coloration, you will obsess about getting there and how you think it appears to others, and you will do everything you can to change the image. If your idealized image is one that is eternally young and free of decay, having heart disease or cancer can be devastating.

In reality, the body is a doorway to bliss. When we learn to open to what the body is always pointing to, we come to realize its transparency and lightness. We can learn to experience the body directly, without the intermediary of memory or anticipation that go to make up its image. For this, we must develop the ability to remain fully open to the current and direct experience of the body. We must learn to notice.

Cultivating the Skill of Noticing

Noticing implies a soft, diffused attention that is inherently nonjudgmental. It is a subtle act of open curiosity, where in a relaxed and loving manner we watch and listen with our whole being. Imagine sitting at a ball game, full of excitement, cheering and booing, the wind and the sun in your face, the ball flying in the air, the crying baby in the bleachers behind you, and your periodic thoughts about work, what to prepare for dinner, or that friend you were supposed to call. Noticing is to take it all in with gentle attentive curiosity without judging any of it or wanting to do anything about it. The heart opener in the previous chapter is a superb exercise in noticing. The most important aspect of noticing is that it is impersonal.

Our conditioning is so strong that it we tend to immediately become entangled with whatever arises in our experience. Almost simultaneously, we start evaluating, judging, comparing, interpreting, or analyzing the experience instead of noticing. As we have seen throughout this book, these mind activities arise from the superhighways that we have built and fortified throughout our lives. As soon as our eyes land on a tree, we name it as oak or maple—and, in the process, we lose the ability to rest in the act of seeing.

Once we become adept at standing as awareness, we can unhook attention from experiencing to simply being. Noticing is subtle because it is not the noticing of something that we are discussing here. It is the act of noticing by being fully open to experience. It is to rest as the noticer of experience. This process results in a shift from the default mode network of the brain that is responsible for our constant autobiographical ruminations to the task positive network, which is engaged in the task at hand. It is a rewiring process for the brain that reveals the secret to finding bliss in the mass of cells that we call the body.

Sensing the Body

In this exercise we will explore the body in a new way. The relaxation induced in this exercise helps to release deeply held contractions in the body. If you find yourself falling asleep midway through this exercise, it is perfectly all right. Most of us are so chronically sleep deprived that the release of tensions aids the descent of deep and restful sleep. Practice this at least a few times a week, and before long you will be able to complete the exercise. You can record this exercise in your own voice, speaking slowly and allowing plenty of time between steps, and use the recording as a guided exercise. Alternatively, you can access this exercise on my website, kavithamd.com.

Exercise: **Sensing the Body**

- Lie down on the floor or a firm bed. You can lie on your back (or on your side if lying on your back is uncomfortable).

- Make yourself as comfortable as possible. Use a pillow under your head and one under your knees if needed. Use an eye pillow or mask and a blanket if you're cold. You have to be able to lie still for 30–45 minutes, so take the time to arrange yourself.

- Take a few deep breaths, prolonging inhalation and exhalation progressively. With each exhalation, see if you can relax a bit more.

- Allow your body to sink into the floor or bed. It is holding you; you don't have to hold up your body. Let gravity do its work.

- Feel the heaviness of your head. Are you holding it up? Let it drop into your pillow. Let go of control over your head and neck.

- Let your shoulders be heavy. They don't need your help while you're lying down. Allow them to drop into the floor or bed. Let your arms follow your shoulders, sinking heavily into the floor or bed.

- Feel the heaviness of your hips and legs as they sink into the surface. Let go of any control over them.

- Allow your back to plop fully into the surface. Feel your entire torso stretching over the surface and burrowing into it.

- Relax fully for a few moments. Bring your attention to your breath. What does the air feel like as you inhale? Can you feel it in your nose and throat without thoughts and images of your nose or throat? Can you feel the sensation of movement as your chest and belly move? What does expansion feel like? How does it feel when the chest and belly contract? If thoughts and images about breathing come up, gently move your attention back to the sensations of breathing.

- Bring your attention to the soles of your feet. Without the image of what they look like, how do you experience the soles of your feet? Notice the sensations of the soles of your feet, such as tingling or pulsing energy. If stories or images come up, gently return to feeling the sensation(s). Does it have a color or texture? Without the image of your feet, can you tell where the sensation is? Does it have a boundary? Without the image of your body, is there an inside and outside to the experience of this sensation? Is there space around it? Simply notice. If thoughts, judgments, evaluations, and interpretations of the sensation come up, gently return to the actual experience of sensing.

- Move your attention in sequence to your ankles, lower legs, knees, thighs, hips, pelvis, lower belly, lower back, upper belly, mid back, chest, upper back, shoulders, upper arms, lower arms, hands, neck, and head. Pause long enough at each point to really feel into the sensations without being caught up in the image of the body part. What does your left hip feel like without your stories and ideas about it? What are your hands without your image of them? Feel into the sensation by becoming curious about its pattern, texture, location, and any space around it.

- Relax for several moments. Without focusing on any particular part of the body, become attentive to all of your experience. Notice the sounds in the room, sensations arising in your body, thoughts, memories, and emotions. Apply the same technique as above— where is it occurring? What does it feel like? Does it have a texture? Is there space around it? Without an image of your body, is there an inside and an outside? Where would that boundary be? What does the boundary arise as? Where? Is there space around it?

- Relax for as long as you need. To end the practice, wiggle your toes and fingers, paying attention to the sensations. Take a few deep breaths, stretching your arms and legs with each inhale and exhaling fully. Support yourself with your arms and sit up.

Deep relaxation and release can have many effects. As the layers of contraction in the physical body are released, there is a growing sense of ease and well-being, increased joyfulness, and a general sense of playfulness about life. At the same time, you must realize that the body is where we hold deep emotional hurts and wounds. As you learn to relax deeply, the channels carrying prana in the subtle body open up, often with a big *whoosh*. Previously stagnant prana is finally able to move through opening channels. This can open up the emotional hurts that are buried under the stagnation and bring them to the surface.

When this happens, realize that it is a good thing! This is the perfect substrate for self-inquiry. Work through the issues using the systematic processes of self-inquiry from chapter 16. Writing down your feelings and thoughts can help bring clarity for self-inquiry. This is why it helps to become at least somewhat acquainted with self-inquiry before moving into the kind of deep body work that we are exploring here in this chapter. With a stable foundation of inner silence cultivated through meditation and the ability to question our inner processes through self-inquiry, we can bravely venture into the process of releasing tightly held beliefs in the body that keep us from fully realizing bliss.

Finding Space in the Body

In the ordinary way of being, the body appears dense because we are unable to sense the spaciousness that is inherent in it. In this exercise we will find the space that pervades the body, within which all sensations occur.

Exercise: Finding Space in the Body

- Perform this exercise in the lying-down position immediately following the sensing the body exercise above.

- Feel the space in front of you. Allow it to fill up the front of your body.

- Feel the space behind you. Allow it to fill up the back of your body.

- Feel the space to the left of your body. Allow it to fill up the left side of your body.

- Feel the space to the right of your body. Allow it to fill up the right side of your body.

- Feel the space in your head, chest, belly, and limbs, slowly proceeding through each part of the body as in the sensing the body exercise above.

- Is there a boundary between the edges of your body and the space around you? If so, what does it feel like?

- Notice that the feeling of a boundary is a sensation. All sensations occur in space. Even the sensation of a boundary arises in space.

- Tune in to the sounds in the room. Where do they occur? Notice that all sensations arise in boundary-less space, whether they are of your own body or of the world around you.

When we learn to tune in to the spaciousness that is in and around our bodies, deeply held contractions loosen up and unwind. We begin to touch the emptiness of our bodies, and the heaviness that previously defined us begins to drop away. Allow this spaciousness to become your new way of being through constant practice. Eventually your body will bloom into a vibrancy and aliveness that you have never known before. From this vantage point, the world will appear different, and your relationship with your body, health, and disease will be one of joy, freedom, and bliss.

Noticing in Movement

The following exercise is meant to open us to noticing while being engaged in movement. Find a place to walk, be it in your living room, backyard, neighborhood, or the woods. Wear comfortable clothing and shoes. You can create your own recording of this exercise and play it as you walk. You can also access it on my website, kavithamd.com.

Exercise: **Noticing in Movement**

- Start walking at an easy pace.

- With each step, allow your foot to sink deeply into the ground. Notice the sensation of contact between the ground and your foot. If you can, pause and close your eyes to sense into the pressure. Where is it? What does it feel like? Without your image of a foot, what does the sensation feel like?

- Bring your attention to the sensations in your ankle, calf, knee, thigh, and hip, focusing on each of these parts with every step. Where are the sensations? Without your ideas and concepts about these body parts, what do they really feel like?

- Bring your attention to your lower belly, upper belly, and chest. What sensations arise as you walk? Simply notice, without evaluation or interpretation of the sensations as good or bad or ideas about why they are happening.

- Bring your attention to your shoulders and arms as you walk. Notice the sensations arising as your whole body engages in walking.

- Walk as long as you need to, paying nonpersonal and nonjudgmental attention to all the sensations arising with each step.

- Notice the objects around you as you walk. Take in the sights, smells, and sounds. What does seeing feel like? Can you sense the process of seeing itself without becoming engaged in the object that the eyes see? What do hearing and smelling feel like? Become interested in the process of sensing without getting engaged in evaluating, interpreting, or judging what you see, hear, or smell. Open fully to the process of noticing without specific focus on objects.

- You can end the practice by sitting or lying down with a brief relaxation, as in the previous exercise.

If you have a yoga posture practice or go to a studio, use these principles while engaged in it. Feel the sensations of movement, balance, and strength in each pose, noticing the spaciousness within which they arise and subside. Notice the sensations in your hands and feet making contact with the floor, the movements of your chest and belly as you breathe, your heartbeats and the space around each.

When we bring stillness and space into movement, we engage with the world in a different way. Sensations become vibrant and scintillating, allowing us to fully immerse ourselves in the experience of what is, rather than the inner commentary about them. Living this way is a great paradox that one of my teachers, Yogani, calls "stillness in action."

Noticing in Daily Life

Once you get used to the lying-down practice, you will develop the ability to notice as you go about your life. One of the most effective ways to rewire our neurohormonal pathways is to put our attention in the body and away from the ruminations of the mind. When you feel stressed or anxious, pause and pay attention to the sensations in the body. Where is this stress? What does it feel like in the body? Does it have a color or texture? Is there space around it? What is the breath doing? Can you feel your heartbeat? What does that feel like? Simply notice the sensations without getting involved in stories and thoughts about them. Just like we learn to gently bring our attention back to the mantra in deep meditation, we learn to gently bring our attention back again and again to the sensation from mental ruminations about them.

When you get upset about a relationship or situation, become curious about what this feels like in your body. What does your breath feel like? Can you feel your heartbeat? What is your reaction presenting itself as in your body? Where is it? Does it have a color or texture? Is there space around it?

When you are sitting in your car or at work, notice what your posture feels like. Tune in to the sensations of your body as you walk from the parking lot to your office. What does the sensation of speaking feel like? Can you sense into the sound of your voice? What do the sensations of taste, smell, hearing, and touch feel like? Can you set aside what you are seeing, tasting, smelling, hearing, and touching and pay attention to the process?

Working with Triggers

One of the most challenging things to work with on this path is the automatic visceral response that comes built-in with our neurohormonal superhighways. We don't even have to wait for a stimulus to complete itself—the response has already begun. If you've ever tried to quit a habit like smoking, you might be able to appreciate the power of this visceral response. Say you've quit smoking recently and are still struggling with the impulse to light up. The slightest stress is enough to override your good intentions—a child's unusual tantrum or a temporary setback at work might trigger the visceral response to smoke with such intensity that it is easier to give in to it than fight it.

The visceral response—be it to smoking, alcohol, sugar, or to particular people, words, and situations—comes about from the well-established nerve connections in the limbic system and the ANS. Our triggers show up in the body as the familiar sensations of discomfort, heart racing, the pit in the stomach, and so on. When it comes to interactions with others, we barely need to listen to what they are saying. Their posture, facial expressions, and tone of voice are enough to trigger the visceral response to such an extent that we are combating with them even before they open their mouth!

Overcoming our visceral responses is hard work. It takes patience and diligence to undo the stubborn pathways in the brain and body. In the following exercise we will explore ways to work with our triggers. Think of a particular trigger that you would like to work with.

Exercise: Working with Triggers

- Perform this exercise in the lying-down position immediately following the sensing the body exercise above.

- In a completely relaxed state, bring up the trigger. It can be the uncontrolled rage or irritation that comes up when your in-law comments on your cooking, the reaction you have when you observe your boss's face when they talk to you, an email you got last night that bothered you, and so on. Allow the trigger to surface.

- Where in the body do you feel it? What do the sensations feel like? Do they have colors or textures? Is there space around them? If justifying, countering, explaining, or interpreting thoughts come up, gently revert your attention to the sensations. Stay entirely with the physical sensations and ignore the mental processes associated with them.

- Notice the process of noticing. What happens when you are genuinely and lovingly curious about how your triggers manifest in your body? Can you find the space in which other responses are possible?

- Stay as long as you need in this contemplation and end the practice as in the sensing the body exercise above.

Once you get a feel for noticing your triggers, you can start practicing in "real life." Let's go back to the example of smoking cessation. You have quit recently and are still struggling with the impulse to light up. *Bam!* The trigger hits you.

- Slow down. Stop whatever you are doing and take two slow and deep breaths. If you can, close your eyes.

- Notice the sensation of the trigger. Where is it? Does it have a color or texture? Does it have a border? Return to the sensation whenever thoughts about it come up. Remain purely with the sensation(s) in the body.

- Notice the space around the sensation. Is there a boundary to this space? Where is it? What does it feel like?

- What happens to the sensation as you continue to notice? Does it move? Where? What does it feel like in the new location?

- Become curious about the process of noticing.

- Can you allow the sensation to be as it is without trying to change it or fix it through a cigarette? Is there another way to respond to this sensation? Can you find that response?

When we slow down and put our attention on the sensations of the trigger, we find that we have innumerable ways to respond and that we are not tied to the same old reaction. Simply allowing the sensation to be as-is frees us from its tyranny. As we progress in these noticing practices, we will find that no sensation is permanent. All sensations come and go, constantly changing and evolving even as we notice them. The sensations of the visceral response are no different. The sensations of the heart racing, the contraction in the stomach, and the inner discomfort instigated by the trigger feel like they are in control because of their urgency that we are unable to bear.

As you will see the very first time you practice this technique, the sensations induced by the trigger eventually abate and subside if you just allow them to be as-is without trying to modify them. The urgency of the sensations can bring up a sense of fear. If this happens, simply notice the sensations of fear. Where are they? What do they feel like?

Noticing is the antidote to the automaticity of triggers. If you can slow down to notice them, you will find that there are other ways to respond to your spouse, boss, or children, the situations that cause your stress in daily life, as well as your addictions.

Working with Pain

One of the greatest blocks to discovering our nature as bliss is identification with physical pain. When we are in pain, it takes over our identity and clouds our perception until it is relieved. Some of this is a natural physiological response—pain is unpleasant and universally unwanted. However, pain is also mostly unavoidable, particularly as we age or when we are afflicted with chronic illnesses. Quite often, chronic pain becomes the story of our lives, where all our interactions with the world are colored by it. With assigning it truth and value (see chapter 16), we make it our identity, the result of which is suffering.

Pain and suffering are two separate issues. We can be in pain but not suffer from it. Suffering is the result of the emotional, social, cultural, and psychological components of pain, which is entirely physical. Pain becomes suffering when we mistake our image of the body to be the body. When we learn to open to the sensation of pain through noticing, a miraculous shift begins to take place. The pain loses its place as the slave master and is seen through for what it is—a conglomeration of sensations and nothing more.

You can try this exercise if you have any pain anywhere in the body. Try it when you have a headache, for instance, or an injury. If you have chronic pain, this exercise will help tremendously to reduce the suffering you might associate with it. The pain might also lessen in intensity or go away. Even if it doesn't, it will not have the same effect on you.

Exercise: Working with Pain

- Perform this exercise in the lying-down position immediately following the sensing the body exercise above.

- In a completely relaxed state, bring your attention to the sensation of the pain. Here we will use the example of knee pain from arthritis. Notice the sensation without the image of the knee. If you get caught up in the story of how much your knee hurts, what your doctor said about it, how it affects your walking, how you wish it was gone, whether you must try another approach, and so on, gently revert your attention to the sensation. What does it feel like without the label of "pain"? Where is it without the image or thought of a knee? Does it have a color or texture? Is there space around it? Notice that the sensation is pure and devoid of all labels and images. Become interested in the process of noticing.

- Does noticing have any boundaries? Does the process of noticing have any pain? What is doing the noticing? Rest here for as long as you want.

- Use this exercise while you are in motion. Without your stories about the pain, what does it feel like while you are walking? Simply notice without evaluation, judgment, or interpretation.

- Notice the spaciousness in which the sensation occurs. You are what is noticing—spacious, blissful, and unaffected by all that occurs in you.

Working with Illness

Having a chronic illness is much like having chronic pain. Even when it is not causing physical pain, illness can become our identity and the way in which we define ourselves. Our naturally spacious bodies become dense and contracted when we believe that illness is the cause of our suffering.

We can work with illness much in the same way as with chronic pain, feeling into the sensations in the body without mind-created images and labels about it. What does heart disease feel like? Set aside your knowledge about how or why it happens, why it should not have happened or how you desperately want to be free of it—these are mental evaluations that have nothing to do with the actual sensations. When they do come up, notice what the associated sensations are like. Where is the anxiety? What does it feel like? Simply notice the sensations. Can you notice the spaciousness in which these sensations arise? What does the process of noticing feel like? What is doing the noticing?

As we work with our bodies in this loving and attentive manner, we begin to see that sensations are delightful arisings in the spaciousness of noticing. We learn to take a step back from the stories that keep us engaged in resistance to sensation and to allow them to be as-is. We do nothing to change them, being completely content with the process of noticing.

With this practice the body becomes light and transparent. It loses the density and heaviness that previously defined it, and instead of seeing it as a mass of flesh and bones, we begin to see it as a spaciousness in which sensations arise and subside. Instead of identifying with the sensations, we begin to see that the spaciousness of noticing is who we really are. We stop taking pain, illness, decay, or death seriously. Decay and death mean nothing without their associated labels and stories that are based in memory; they have no basis in current experience. We become established in the process as it is occurring now, interested at all times in being here now.

Summary

- We experience the body in a certain way because we have an image of it. Over time, this image becomes so embedded in our psyche that we start taking the image to be the body.

- Noticing implies a soft, diffused attention that is inherently nonjudgmental. It is a subtle act of open curiosity, where we watch and listen with our whole being in a relaxed and loving manner.

- As we learn to relax deeply, the channels carrying prana in the subtle body open up, and emotional hurts that are buried under the stagnation can be brought up to the surface. Self-inquiry is then employed to work with the arising issues.

- As we work with our bodies in a loving and attentive manner, we begin to see that sensations are delightful arisings in the spaciousness of noticing. We learn to take a step back from the stories that keep us engaged in resistance to sensation and to allow them to be as-is. We do nothing to change them, being completely content with the process of noticing.

Conclusion

Living Bliss

If you've followed along thus far, you may have wondered where it might eventually lead. This is a valid question with no straight answer since there is no end goal to this journey. Because of the infinite nature of bliss, there is no end point that we can possibly reach.

As you continue to practice the steps of the bliss Rx, you will learn to access the stillness and peace of the here and now with increasing effortlessness. When you start becoming interested in the process of noticing, you will open to the inherent sweetness and bliss of your true nature. You start to become increasingly established in the bliss of self-awareness. With this, your life will continue as before, but nothing will be the same.

You may still have your chronic illness or the issues of daily life, but your relationship with them has changed. You are neither avoiding them nor rejecting them but allowing them to be. You love life as it is and don't have an agenda because you are steeped in contentment and peace. Fear, cravings, and insecurity are things of the past. When you realize that you are not your body-mind, your own thoughts make no sense to you. When you stop paying attention to your thoughts and taking them seriously, they eventually stop arising. When this happens, you become the master of your mind, using it to do creative work, for planning and organizing, and for solving problems. When not engaged in this functional way, the mind rests in silence without the constant chatter and narration that marked your previous state of being. It has no control over you.

When your mind loses control over you, you are free from its evaluations, interpretations, judgments, and comparisons. Your neurohormonal pathways have slowed down, and your visceral responses no longer carry an emotional charge. You start to see the world for what it is: vibrant, colorful, and beautiful. You see that the only truth to any experience is the experience itself. All meanings are functions of conditioning and how we have forged our neurohormonal superhighways.

Instead of trying to cultivate the virtues of gratitude, compassion, and forgiveness from the outside-in, we are pleasantly surprised to see that these virtues are inherent in our true nature. When we work to redo our own neurohormonal superhighways, we find that these qualities of interactions with others had been within us all along. With the parting of the veil of conditioning, these qualities radiate out from the bliss of our own true nature. We find that we have always been home.

Traversing the Path

Living bliss is a gradual and incremental process. It can take years to reforge our neurohormonal superhighways because they are so deeply etched in our subtle bodies. Initially, it can be shocking when we become aware of our processes. We might realize how selfish our actions seem, how conniving our mind is, how fearful and judgmental our thoughts are. The beauty of this process is that becoming aware of our patterns is healing in itself. Brought to light, these instincts squirm like fish out of water. They dissolve as we continue to observe them, and the underlying wisdom shines through.

The peculiar thing about this path is that once you commit to it, it will pull you in all the way. Even if you take a break or discontinue the program, the path will find you in another way. If the practices of the bliss Rx don't appeal to you but your interest is gripped by the path, it will find you another resource, teacher, or book that will lead you to the beauty and bliss of your true nature. Your life will become a stream of miracles, with synchronicities and events that propel you along the path.

The path will light itself in such a way that one day, you will turn around and see that your entire life has been a stream of miracles. Not a single event in your life has been accidental, including picking up this book. At every moment you were given exactly what you needed to wake up to the beauty of your own nature. When you turn back around and take your next step, you can rest assured that it will be perfect. You are perfect, flawless, and whole.

Glossary

Acetylcholine. The neurotransmitter responsible for the rest-and-digest response.

Acute Coronary Syndrome. Heart attack.

Agni. The fire of transformation in nature, body, and mind.

Alpha Waves. Brain waves seen in relaxation and focus, ranging from 8–12 Hz.

Ama. The toxic residue of incomplete digestion resulting from an imbalanced agni.

Angina. Chest discomfort that may indicate heart disease.

Angioplasty. Opening the artery without surgery by inserting a balloon into the blocked area and inflating it.

Ardha Siddhasana. Half of siddhasana (see below).

Arteries. Blood vessels leaving the heart.

Atherosclerosis. The hardening of the arteries that results in blockages.

Autonomic Nervous System (ANS). Part of the peripheral nervous system that is out of our voluntary control.

Ayurveda. The ancient medical science that translates as "science of life."

Beta Waves. Brain waves seen during waking hours, ranging from 12–38 Hz.

Bhakti Yoga. The path of devotion.

Causal Body. Made of impressions and drives the physical and subtle bodies as actions, choices and thoughts.

Central nervous system (CNS). Part of the nervous system consisting of the brain and the spinal cord.

Chakras. Energy centers of the subtle body that are seen as wheels in the mind's eye when activated.

Chromosomes. Thread-like structures in the nucleus of the cell that become most obvious just before a cell divides, containing DNA.

Chronobiology. The study of internal clocks and their relationship to disease and health.

Coronary Arteries. Blood vessels that supply oxygen and nutrients to the heart.

Default Mode Network (DMN). Network of various brain centers that light up simultaneously when focused attention is not required.

Delta Waves. Brain waves in deep, dreamless sleep, ranging from 0.5-3 Hz

DNA. Deoxyribonucleic acid, the carrier of genetic material.

Dopamine. Hormone that makes us seek pleasure.

Doshas. The three main principles or energies that go on to create the structure and functioning of the universe, including our body-mind.

Endorphins. Hormones that make us feel good.

Epigenetics. The study of environmental factors that turn genes on or off without altering the underlying DNA sequence.

Estrogen. Hormone responsible for differences between male and female brains and behavior.

Gamma Waves. Brain waves in blissful states, ranging from 38–42 Hz.

Gunas. The three universal qualities of creation. See also *rajas, sattva,* and *tamas.*

Hawthorne Effect. The phenomenon where the behavior of individuals being observed changes when they are aware that they are being watched.

HDL. High-density lipoprotein, a type of cholesterol.

Holism. Theory which states that the universe and especially living nature is correctly seen in terms of interacting wholes that are more than the mere sum of elementary particles.

Kapha. The principle of structure, heaviness, and stability.

Karma Yoga. The path of selfless service.

LDL. Low-density lipoprotein, a type of cholesterol.

Nadis. The energy channels of the subtle body that carry our life force.

Neuroplasticity. The ability of the brain to change based on experience and outlook.

Norepinephrine. The neurotransmitter responsible for the flight-or-fight response.

Observer Effect. The phenomenon where observing something changes its outcome.

Ojas. The subtle essence of kapha, the vital reserve of the body.

Oscillators. Clock mechanisms in major organ systems including the liver, heart, kidneys, and skeletal muscles.

Oxytocin. Hormone that makes us feel attachment and form bonds with others.

Pitta. The dosha responsible for transformation and metabolism.

Prana. The essential life force that enables the functioning of our body-mind.

Pranayama. Regulation of prana through regulating the breath.

Psychoneuroimmunology (PNI). Branch of science that incorporates psychology, behavioral science, neuroscience, immunology, physiology, endocrinology, genetics, genomics, and other sciences.

Rajas. The guna of movement, dynamism, change, and activity.

Sattva. The guna of intelligence, lightness, contentment, and sweetness.

Serotonin. Hormone that makes us feel good in comparison with others.

Siddhasana. Perfected pose. A posture for meditation.

Subtle Body. Made up of energy, mind, and intellect.

Suprachiasmatic Nuclei (SCN). The master clock of the body.

Tamas. The guna of structure, heaviness, inertia, and stagnation.

Tejas. The subtle essence of pitta, the quality of light, heat, and radiance.

Telomeres. Protective caps at the end of chromosomes.

Theta Waves. Brain waves seen in deep meditation, ranging from 3–8 Hz.

Vata. The principle of dryness, coolness, and movement.

Vedanta. A path of spiritual practice where we come to realize our true nature as awareness through logic and inquiry.

Veins. Blood vessels coming to the heart.

Yoga. A path of spiritual practice where we seek self-realization as the union of our lower self (body-mind) with our higher self (awareness).

Zeitgebers. External influences of the SCN, the master clock.

Resources

Holistic Heart Health

Kahn, J. *The Whole Heart Solution: Halt Heart Disease Now with the Best Alternative and Traditional Medicine.* The Reader's Digest Association, 2013.

Ornish, D. *Dr. Dean Ornish's Program for Reversing Heart Disease: The Only System Scientifically Proven to Reverse Heart Disease without Drugs or Surgery.* Random House, 1990.

Schneider, R. H., and J. Z. Fields. *Total Heart Health: How to Prevent and Reverse Heart Disease with the Maharishi Vedic Approach to Health.* Basic Health Publications, 2006.

Sinatra, S. T., and M. C. Houston. American College of Nutrition (U.S.) *Nutritional and Integrative Strategies in Cardiovascular Medicine.* CRC Press, Taylor & Francis Group, 2015.

Science and Biology

Breuning, L. G. *Habits of a Happy Brain.* Adams Media, 2015.

Feuerstein, G. *The Psychology of Yoga: Integrating Eastern and Western Approaches for Understanding the Mind.* Shambhala, 2013.

Lipton, B. H. *The Biology of Belief: Unleashing the Power of Consciousness, Matter & Miracles.* Hay House, 2015.

Science and Nonduality website: https://www
.scienceandnonduality.com/

Van der Kolk, B. A. *The Body Keeps the Score: Brain, Mind, and Body in the Healing of Trauma.* Viking, 2014.

Ayurveda/Holistic Health

Borysenko, J. *Minding the Body, Mending the Mind.* Da Capo, 2007.

Chaudhary, K. *The Prime: Prepare and Repair Your Body for Spontaneous Weight Loss.* Harmony, 2016.

Chopra, D. *Quantum Healing: Exploring the Frontiers of Mind/Body Medicine.* Bantam, 2015.

Fondin, M. S. *The Wheel of Healing with Ayurveda: An Easy Guide to a Healthy Lifestyle.* New World Library, 2015.

Frawley, D. *Ayurvedic Healing: A Comprehensive Guide.* Lotus Press, 2001.

Kshirsagar, S. G., and D. Chopra. *The Hot Belly Diet: A 30-Day Ayurvedic Plan to Reset Your Metabolism, Lose Weight, and Restore Your Body's Natural Balance to Heal Itself.* Atria, 2015.

Lad, V. *The Complete Book of Ayurvedic Home Remedies: Based on the Timeless Wisdom of India's 5,000-Year-Old Medical System.* Harmony, 1999.

O' Donnell, K., and C. Brostrom. *The Everyday Ayurveda Cookbook: A Seasonal Guide to Eating and Living Well.* Shambhala, 2015.

Svoboda, R. *Ayurveda: Life, Health, and Longevity.* Ayurvedic Press, 2004.

Tiwari, M. *Ayurveda: A Life of Balance—The Complete Guide to Ayurvedic Nutrition and Body Types with Recipes.* Healing Arts Press, 1995.

Yarema, T., D. Rhoda, and J. Brannigan. *Eat-Taste-Heal: An Ayurvedic Cookbook for Modern Living.* Five Elements Press, 2006.

Women's Health

Lonsdorf, N. *The Ageless Woman: How to Navigate the Transition Naturally for a Long Life of Vibrant Health and Radiant Beauty.* MUM Press, 2016.

Lonsdorf, N., V. Butler, and M. Brown. *A Woman's Best Medicine: Health, Happiness, and Long Life Through Maharishi Ayurveda.* Tarcher Putnam, 1995.

Northrup, C. *Women's Bodies, Women's Wisdom: Creating Physical and Emotional Health and Healing.* Bantam, 2010.

Raichur, P., and M. Cohn. *Absolute Beauty: Radiant Skin and Inner Harmony Through the Ancient Secrets of Ayurveda.* HarperCollins, 1997.

Svoboda, R. *Ayurveda for Women: A Guide to Vitality and Health.* Healing Arts Press, 2000.

Welch, C. *Balance Your Hormones, Balance Your Life: Achieving Optimal Health and Wellness Through Ayurveda, Chinese Medicine, and Western Science.* Da Capo Press, 2011.

Meditation and Pranayama

Bliss Meditation Course: http://kavithamd.com/bliss-meditation-course/

Guided Mindfulness Meditation Practices with Jon Kabat-Zinn: https://www.mindfulnesscds.com/

Transcendental Meditation: https://www.tm.org/

Yogani. *Deep Meditation: Pathway to Personal Freedom.* AYP Publishing, 2005.

———. *Advanced Yoga Practices: Easy Lessons for Ecstatic Living.* AYP Publishing, 2004.

Yogani's Advanced Yoga Practices website: http://aypsite.com/

Decluttering Physical Space

Kondo, M., and C. Hirano. *The Life-Changing Magic of Tidying Up: The Japanese Art of Decluttering and Organizing.* Ten Speed Press, 2014.

Self-Inquiry

Goode, G. *The Direct Path: A User Guide.* Non-Duality, 2012.

Kahn, M. *Whatever Arises, Love That: A Love Revolution that Begins with You.* Sounds True, 2016.

Katie, B., and S. Mitchell. *Loving What Is: Four Questions That Can Change Your Life.* Three Rivers Press, 2003.

Kelly, L. *Shift into Freedom: The Science and Practice of Open-Hearted Awareness.* Sounds True, 2015.

Working with the Body

Doyle, B. *Yoga in the Kashmir Tradition: The Art of Listening.* Non-Duality, 2014.

Kaparo, R. *Awakening Somatic Intelligence: The Art and Practice of Embodied Mindfulness—Transform Pain, Stress, Trauma, and Aging.* North Atlantic Books, 2012.

Index

health in, 29, 35
neurohormonal pathways
and, 89–90
unity in, 33
Bliss Rx, 2–3, 135–142
acceptance and, 20, 22
balancing vata and, 146
building blocks of, 10
clarity of perception and,
225–241
compassion and, 19, 22
decluttering and, 199–211
dietary practices and,
165–181, 182
disclaimer, 11–12
effects and benefits of,
17–21, 22
forgiveness and, 19, 22
goal of, 3, 138
gratitude and, 20, 22
harmony and, 140
inner silence and, 183–196
inside-out approach, *136*,
137
kindling the fire and,
145–161
lifestyle changes and, 18, 22
loss of victimization,
18–19, 22
opening to bliss and,
213–222
origins of, 4–8
outside-in approach,
135–37, *136*
phases of evolution, 139–
142, 143
practicing, 8–9

recipes, 173–78
reduction of stress and, 18, 22
sample meal plan, 179–180
stability and, 141
stagnation and, 140
timelines and, 137–39
trepidation and, 139–140
turmoil and, 140–41
Bliss Spice Mix, 174
Bliss Tea, 173
blood, 38, 39
amount in adults, 52
blood tests, 40, 49
bodies, three, 107–10
body
bliss in the, 243–257
causal, 109, 115, 117, 118,
128, 264
default model and, 25
idealized image of,
243–44, 258
illness and, 257
knowing and, 243–44
no ability to care, 24–25
noticing and, 244–45
noticing in daily life, 251–52
noticing in movement,
250–51
pain and, 255–56
physical, 107, 109, 117, 118,
127–28
relaxation and release, 248
sensing the, 245–48
space in the, 248–49, 257
subtle, 107–9, 117, 118, 128,
213–15, 216–17, 223, 266
triggers and, 252–55